The Growth of Nursing Home Care

The Growth of Nursing Home Care

Burton David Dunlop
The Urban Institute

Lexington Books
D.C. Heath and Company
Lexington, Massachusetts
Toronto

Library of Congress Cataloging in Publication Data

Dunlop, Burton D.
   The growth of nursing home care.

   Includes index.
   1. Nursing homes—United States. 2. Nursing homes—United States—Utilization. 3. Nursing homes—United States—Finance. I. Title.
RA997.D86   362.6'11'6   78-14715
ISBN 0-669-02704-9

The work upon which this monograph is based was performed pursuant to Contract No. HEW-100-76-0069 between The Urban Institute and the Office of the Secretary, U.S. Department of Health, Education and Welfare. The views expressed here are those of the author and do not necessarily reflect those of HEW, The Urban Institute, or its sponsors.

Published simultaneously in Canada.

Printed in the United States of America.

International Standard Book Number: 0-669-02704-9

Library of Congress Catalog Card Number: 78-14715

To Sandi, my wife, and to Kimberly and Kristin, my daughters, who patiently endured the many hours I was occupied in carrying out the research and in writing up the results reported here.

Contents

List of Figures

List of Tables

Foreword

Long-term care has become a central issue for those interested in the welfare of impaired elderly and other disabled groups in this country. Many are convinced that the present number of long-term care facilities is not adequate to meet the needs of these groups. At the same time, legislators and the heads of federal and state agencies are becoming increasingly alarmed over the rising cost of publicly financed long-term care. They note that in 1976 the Medicaid program spent $5 billion on nursing home care, representing 40 percent of the total Medicaid budget. In recent years the Department of Health, Education and Welfare has set up several long-term care task forces to develop policy options in this area. To date, such efforts have not resulted in any specific legislative proposal. It should also be noted that none of the major national health insurance bills receiving serious consideration by Congress includes long-term care coverage.

The reluctance to address long-term care in national health insurance planning seems to be caused by the uncertainties of program cost. How would the availability of publicly funded in-home care be controlled to avoid abuse? How would nonmedically oriented facilities—that is, domiciliary care homes and other supportive residential environments—be involved in a new system? Would a greater supply of such facilities induce people to use them?

The concern seems related to the widespread belief that the growth in the supply of nursing homes was caused by the greater availability of funding under Medicare and Medicaid. This, combined with the fact that occupancy rates in nursing homes have historically been very high, has led a number of health planners to conclude that supply induces demand in the long-term care area. As a result, some states have placed some form of restriction on the construction of nursing homes.

The study conducted by Dr. Dunlop on the growth in the supply of nursing home beds between the mid-1960s and the mid-1970s provides considerable insight into some of these important policy issues. First, there is strong reason to doubt that Medicaid financing accelerated the growth of nursing homes. Significant demand elements appear to have exerted considerable impact quite independently of financial incentives to nursing home owners. Secondly, actions taken to hold down nursing home costs and to deter nursing home expansion have contributed to the placement of some people in more costly facilities than necessary, while others are denied access to facilities when, in fact, they require such care.

Throughout this report, the connection between medical services and social services in the provision of long-term care is emphasized. Understanding this relationship is essential for comprehensive long-term care planning. Another contribution of this study is its focus on the interrelationships of long-term care arrangements. Nursing homes are only one component of long-term care.

Subsidies and regulations that affect the supply and demand for nursing home care have consequences for general hospitals, mental hospitals, formal in-home services, and supportive residential facilities, as well as for families. Dr. Dunlop makes specific policy recommendations for dealing with some of these consequences and suggests areas where additional information should be gathered in order to more completely understand the long-term care continuum.

August 1, 1978   *Jeffrey J. Koshel, Director*
                                                    Social Services Research Program
                                                    The Urban Institute

Acknowledgments

Many individuals deserve credit for the successful completion of the study reported here. The contributions of several present and former colleagues at The Urban Institute are especially noteworthy.

Special thanks go first of all to William Pollak, whose contributions were many. In managing the study project over the first eight months, he was largely responsible for shaping the study approach. He also formulated a number of the tables used here and wrote much of the sample selection description contained in appendix E. Jane Weeks and Lydia Skloven provided valuable research assistance in the data compilation and processing tasks. Jane Weeks also researched and wrote up the details of federal policies since 1950, many of which appear here as appendix B. William Scanlon and John Holahan took the time to provide helpful comments on an early draft of this book. Jeffrey Koshel supplied very valuable direction throughout the study and the writing of many drafts.

I am also very much indebted to all the health, welfare, social service, and nursing home association officials (too many to name) in Alabama, California, Florida, Mississippi, New Jersey, New York, South Dakota, Vermont, West Virginia, and Wisconsin who provided data and who took time to explain the intricacies of eligibility, reimbursement, licensure, capital subsidy, and planning policies in their respective states. Without their assistance, the central question of what role state and federal policies played in nursing home growth over the study period could not have been addressed.

None of the above, of course, bears any responsibility for errors, omissions, or misinterpretations that may exist in this book. That responsibility rests with the author alone.

1 Introduction

It seems that barely a day passes without some national media source devoting significant attention to nursing homes in the United States. Often the coverage involves alleged abuse of either patients or public monies in this largely proprietary industry. Nursing homes have become very visible parts of the institutional and health care landscape in this country. This visibility, however, is a relatively recent phenomenon.

It is widely perceived that use of nursing homes in this country has grown dramatically over the past few years. Indeed, between 1963 and 1973 the number of nursing home beds in the nation grew from 510,180 to 1,107,358 beds—an overall increase of 117 percent and an average annual expansion rate of 8.1 percent. Over that same period, the number of nursing home beds per 100 elderly population rose 80 percent, from 2.9 to 5.2.

Understandably, increases in expenditures for nursing home care, especially those made by government, have been equally dramatic. National expenditures for nursing home care in FY 1963 totaled $891.0 million. By 1973 they had risen to $6.7 billion. Public expenditures by 1973 had reached $3.2 billion, while in 1963 they came to only $337.0 million.

The increased supply and utilization of long-term care has been attributed to a number of factors. Among others, these include advances in biomedicine which have allowed a much larger number of persons to survive to ages at which increasing impairments impose the need for care, increased population mobility and sociocultural changes which lessen the likelihood that family will provide care, increased public financing of institutional care which broadens access, and improved quality of nursing home care which may diminish people's reluctance to use nursing homes. The dramatic growth of recent years, however, is most often attributed to the enactment of Medicare and Medicaid.

In light of such heavy increases in both expenditures and use, there is widespread concern that we may be relying too heavily upon nursing homes to care for our impaired elderly population. Consequently, the office of the Assistant Secretary for Planning and Evaluation of the U.S. Department of Health, Education and Welfare sponsored the Nursing Home Supply and Demand Study. The study objectives were to identify those factors accounting for nursing home growth and, in particular, to determine what role governmental programs played in such growth over the period 1964-1974.

This monograph reports on the findings of one of the major parts of that overall study effort—a series of case study analyses of nursing home policies and growth patterns in ten states.

1

Major Findings

Major findings from these research efforts include the following:

> Growth in nursing home bed stock was more rapid before the implementation of Medicaid and Medicare than afterward. Rapid growth occurring in the mid-1960s was a continuation of a pattern of increasing growth that appears to have begun with the adoption of federal vendor payment programs in the 1950s and early 1960s.
>
> Contrary to popular impression, Medicaid and Medicare did not represent some kind of "quantum leap" in public nursing home care policy. The size of Medicare funding has been quite small and has been limited to coverage of short-term, posthospital recuperation. Medicaid, in large measure, was a replacement funding source for earlier medical assistance programs and brought little change overall in eligibility determination. These programs do appear to have enabled the continuation of an established pattern of rapid growth through their encouragement of more generous reimbursement levels, however, and to have brought widespread enforcement of nursing home standards for the first time.
>
> Again, despite widely publicized scandals and rather numerous and impassioned indictments of the nursing home industry in recent years, the image of nursing home care among physicians, caseworkers, and the general population appears to have improved markedly—relative to the image prevalent in the early 1960s—as a result of the greatly enhanced enforcement of nursing home standards. This development, in itself, thus appears to have contributed to demand for nursing home beds in recent years.
>
> Although no single factor can account for the growth in the demand for nursing home care, our analysis indicates that the very dramatic increase over the past decade or two in the number of very old elderly—especially unmarried females—who tend to suffer reduced physical, social, and economic resources with which to maintain independence is the single most important development.
>
> A second important factor increasing demand is the substitution of nursing home care for that formerly delivered in other settings—principally mental institutions and also general hospitals. Nursing homes have become the dominant long-term care mode in this country, in large part, because of the direction of federal subsidies.
>
> Nursing home bed supply has not kept pace with demand for nursing home care. With the exception of a few localities, a state of chronic excess demand has characterized the nursing home market throughout the study period. This state of affairs has exacerbated a number of problems for

policymakers, including inappropriate placement, ineffectual needs assessment, and weakened standards enforcement. A decrease in the rate of growth of the older elderly population in the 1970s may contribute to less intense demand in the immediate future. On the other hand, state efforts to control Medicaid costs, including limitations on capital expansion of the nursing home bed stock, may perpetuate the bed shortage.

Summary of Policy Implications

The findings of this study suggest that instead of seeking to effect a larger supply of nursing home beds to meet the heavy demand for long-term care, future governmental efforts would be much more appropriately directed toward expanding the supply of alternatives to nursing home care—especially supportive residential facilities. A significant expansion of alternatives would comprise an important part of the solution to both excess demand and the resulting barriers to enforcement of quality in nursing homes. Along with equitable reimbursement rates according to care level and comprehensive planning for all long-term care settings, expansion of alternatives also seems likely to help in reducing the ineffectiveness of needs assessment and lessening inappropriate placement. With such an expansion, the existing nursing home bed stock level, perhaps with periodic incremental increases, might prove adequate to meet the need for care that truly requires a substantial nursing component.

In-home benefits under Medicare and Medicaid clearly are inadequate to make home care a realistic alternative to nursing homes at present. Substantial liberalization of coverage to include nonmedical care under these programs, under National Health Insurance or under some other mechanism such as the "long-term care center" proposed in a number of recent congressional bills, appears needed in order to make this care setting a viable alternative. Even then, there is no guarantee that such liberalization would reduce the likelihood of nursing home admissions, especially for those significantly impaired persons who lack informal supports.

Economic theory would suggest that the most efficacious way of effecting a larger supply of supportive residential beds is through higher reimbursement. Of note, changes proposed in the Carter Administration's welfare reform package affecting Supplemental Security Income, if enacted, could result in diminished rather than enhanced reimbursement because they appear to remove the federal match incentive under the SSI program for states to supplement the basic cash grant to individuals residing in group homes. The proposed federal income floor alone may be inadequate to purchase care in desirable facilities.

To insure an adequate mix of SNF and ICF level beds, it appears that reimbursement should be tied to relative costs of providing care. If federal mandates to the states to establish cost-related reimbursement determination procedures fail to produce this type of reimbursement structure, some additional federal action may be required.

The foregoing discussion implies that if the provision of long-term care is to be coordinated so that alternative formal care modes emerge, and if long-range costs are to be controlled, certificate-of-need or other comprehensive planning mechanisms should cover all long-term care settings. (Presently, very few states include any long-term care settings other than SNFs and ICFs under their certificate-of-need program as only these are viewed as components of the health care system.)

Finally, the previous discussion implies that the federal posture with regard to supply of nursing home beds versus demand for nursing home care can be most directly realized in the foreseeable future through guidelines, directives, and incentives issued within its health planning programs and through reimbursement or federal cost-sharing policies. Study findings clearly indicate, however, that various policies affecting nursing homes are interactive in their impacts. This means that any proposed policy change should be considered in light of its probable effects on other policy and program areas affecting nursing home care.

Chapter Outline

The next chapter presents a detailed description of the issues addressed by this study. It compares the nursing home growth pattern during different segments of the study period and for proprietary and nonprofit nursing homes. Growth in nursing home expenditures and variations across localities in nursing home utilization levels are noted. Next, variables known or hypothesized to affect nursing home utilization are discussed along with available supporting data. This discussion of hypotheses sets the stage for the direction of analysis to follow.

A full description of the method of analysis employed in this study is provided in chapter 3. As the reader will note, careful thought was given to representativeness of the sample states and hence to the generalizability of findings from those states. Special treatment of data made necessary by limitations on data availability, as well as the relative weight given to each of the data sources in formulating study conclusions, are indicated. In the final section of this chapter, the nursing home growth patterns of the sample states as a whole and of subgroups of sample states are discussed and compared with the growth pattern for the country. Review of this section will provide the reader with a better sense of the generalizability of findings from the case studies.

Chapter 4 is concerned with sociodemographic and institutional developments during the last decade or two that increased the demand for nursing home services among the elderly population. The age structure of the elderly population is given particularly close attention. Other sociodemographic changes are suggested as probable influences on increased utilization of nursing home care for all age brackets among the elderly. This chapter then moves into a discussion of the impact on nursing home use of deinstitutionalization of mental hospitals and of the substitution of nursing home care for that formerly rendered in general hospitals, in supportive residential settings, and even at home. These developments have helped to make nursing homes the dominant formal setting for the delivery of long-term care in this country.

In chapter 5, the programs through which federal and state governments have subsidized nursing home care are analyzed for their impacts on expanded use and supply of nursing home care over the period 1964-1974. The effects of eligibility determination criteria for nursing home care on demand for nursing home beds are discussed, and an attempt is made to decipher the impacts of various facets of reimbursement policy on the decisions of nursing home operators to expand the bed supply. In the final section of chapter 5 we discuss the role played by capital funding sources, particularly federal subsidies, on nursing home expansion activities over the study period.

Chapter 6 examines the means by which state and federal policymakers have attempted through industry regulation to ensure that subsidies provided are well spent. Considerable attention is focused on the promulgation and enforcement of state licensure and federal certification standards. We attempt to trace the effects of these regulatory efforts both on quality of care and subsequent level of demand and on the bed supply. Specific note is taken of the influence of Hill-Burton standards, issued by the Public Health Service in 1954, on this process. The latter portion of the chapter is devoted to a review of governmental initiatives taken to directly shape and limit the nursing home bed supply.

Because of the special interest of policymakers in the roles that Medicare and Medicaid have played in the rapid nursing home growth observed in recent years, we have set aside chapter 7 for a discussion of the impacts of these programs not only on growth but also on the changing character of nursing home provision in this country. Impacts of Medicaid on eligibility, reimbursement, standards, capital funding, planning, and investment controls are treated separately. Some of the program descriptions presented in earlier chapters are reintroduced here so that they can be better understood in relation to these most recent federal subsidy programs. Because Medicare has played such a minor role compared to other funding mechanisms in the provision of nursing home care over the study period, detailed treatment of the size of Medicare support for long-term care and its impact are limited largely to the last section of this chapter.

In the final chapter of this book, we summarize materials presented in earlier chapters and identify those factors which seem to have been the most important determinants of the rapid expansion in nursing home supply and demand which this country experienced over the study period. This is followed by a delineation of some major problems facing policymakers that have been created or exacerbated by the state of chronic excess demand found in this study to characterize the nursing home industry. The emerging role of planning controls in shaping the nursing home bed supply is also outlined. The chapter continues with a discussion of the policy implications of some of the major study findings, especially the steps needed to ameliorate the nursing home bed shortage and the misalignment of care need and care setting. The book concludes with a brief discussion of those developments that appear most likely to influence nursing home growth in the foreseeable future.

Statement of the Problem

As indicated in chapter 1, the United States has experienced a dramatic growth in the size and visibility of the nursing home industry over the past decade. Over the period 1963 to 1973, as reflected in table 2-1, the number of nursing home beds increased 117 percent and the number of beds per 100 elderly persons rose from 2.9 to 5.2—an 80 percent increase. Between 1963 and 1973, the number of nursing home beds rose at an average annual rate of 8.1 percent, from 510,180 beds in the earlier year to 1,107,358 beds in 1973. Over the same time span the number of facilities increased at an annual rate of only 1.5 percent, from 12,825 to 14,873 (see table 2-2). The much slower growth in the number of facilities relative to the expansion of beds reflects progressive increases in the average size of facilities.

These statistics reflect data compiled by the National Center for Health Statistics. NCHS places nursing homes and related facilities into four categories: Nursing Care Homes, Personal Care Homes with Nursing, Personal Care Homes without Nursing, and Domiciliary Care Homes. The center has undertaken censuses of these facilities in 1963, 1967, 1969, 1971, 1973, and 1976. In this monograph nursing home figures for 1963-1969 reflect the sum of the first two NCHS categories while for 1971 to 1973, figures reflect only the "Nursing Care Home" category. This treatment of NCHS data provides optimal alignment with state licensure data. Fuller treatment of this data alignment concern is provided in appendix C.

The index of nursing home utilization by which growth will be compared in this work is beds per 100 elderly population. Rates of growth relative to the size of the elderly population are meaningful because the aged are by far the dominant users of nursing home care. Approximately 89 percent of the nursing home population is composed of elderly persons. Use of rates per elderly population thus standardizes for this rather uninteresting relationship.

If the bed supply figures are viewed for three separate periods—1963 through 1966, 1967 through 1970, and 1971 to 1973—they reveal a changing growth pattern. Over the earliest period, bed supplies increased at an average annual rate of 10.7 percent; over the middle period the growth of beds slowed to an annual rate of 5.4 percent; and over the third period, growth recovered somewhat to an average annual rate of 8.3 percent. In terms of growth in number of beds per 100 elderly, the nation as a whole experienced an increase of 8.7 percent during the period 1963 through 1966, 3.6 percent during the years 1967 through 1970, and 6.1 percent between 1971 and 1973.

Table 2-1
Number of Beds in Nursing Homes by Ownership Type, 1963-1973

	1963	1964	1967	1969	1971	1973
Total Nursing Home Beds[a]	510,180	556,600	765,148	879,091	944,697	1,107,358
Average Annual Percent Increase—Beds[b]	—	9.1	11.2	7.2	3.6	8.2
Population 65+	17,785,000	18,108,000	19,066,000	19,754,000	20,488,000	21,346,000
Beds per 100 Elderly (65+)	2.87	3.07	4.01	4.45	4.61	5.19
Average Annual Percent Increase—Beds per 100 Elderly[b]	—	7.0	9.3	5.3	1.7	6.1
Number { Proprietary	307,958	344,900	NA[c]	585,284	684,586	754,189
Nonprofit	118,876	132,000		213,947	166,025	247,576
Government	83,346	79,700		79,860	94,086	105,593
Percent of Total { Proprietary	60.4	62.0	NA	66.6	72.5	68.1
Nonprofit	23.3	23.7		24.3	17.6	22.4
Government	16.3	14.3		9.1	10.0	9.5

Sources: DHEW, NCHS, *Utilization of Institutions for the Aged and Chronically Ill: United States—April-June 1963*, February 1966; DHEW, NCHS, *Arrangements for Physician Services to Residents in Nursing and Personal Care Homes: United States—May-June 1964*, February 1970; DHEW, NCHS, *Health Resources Statistics*, May 1970; DHEW, NCHS, *Health Resources Statistics*, February 1972; DHEW, NCHS, *Health Resources Statistics*, 1974; unpublished data from the NCHS Master Facility Census; U.S. Bureau of the Census, *Preliminary Estimates of the Population of the United States, by Age and Sex: April 1, 1960, to July 1, 1971*, Series P-25, No. 483, April 1972; U.S. Bureau of the Census, *Estimates of the Population of the United States, by Age, Sex, and Race: 1970 to 1975*, Series P-25, No. 614, 1975.

[a]For 1963-1969 this figure represents the sum of the NCHS Nursing Care Home and Personal Care Home with Nursing categories; and for 1971 and 1973 the figure represents the Nursing Care Home category alone.

[b]Figures are average annual rates of change from the year of the preceding column to the year for which the figure is shown.

[c]NA = Not Available.

Table 2-2

Number of Nursing Homes by Ownership Type, 1963-1973

		1963	1964	1967	1969	1971	1973
Total Nursing Homes[a]		12,825	14,520	14,489	14,998	13,204	14,873
Percent Increase[b]		–	13.2	–0.1	1.7	–6.2	6.1
Average Size		39.9	38.3	52.8	58.6	71.5	74.5
Proprietary			11,860	11,287	11,508	10,242	10,987
Nonprofit	Number	NA[c]	1,890	2,358	2,628	2,072	2,926
Government			770	844	862	890	960
Proprietary			81.7	77.9	76.7	77.6	73.9
Nonprofit	Percent of Total	NA	13.0	16.3	15.5	15.7	19.7
Government			5.3	5.8	5.8	6.7	6.4
Proprietary			29.1		50.9	66.8	68.6
Nonprofit	Average Size	NA	69.8	NA	81.4	80.1	84.6
Government			103.5		92.6	105.7	110.0

Sources: DHEW, NCHS, *Utilization of Institutions for the Aged and Chronically Ill: United States—April-June 1963,* February 1966; DHEW, NCHS, *Arrangements for Physician Services to Residents in Nursing and Personal Care Homes: United States—May-June 1964,* February 1970; DHEW, NCHS, *Health Resources Statistics,* May 1970; DHEW, NCHS, *Health Resources Statistics,* February 1972; DHEW, NCHS, *Health Resources Statistics,* 1974; unpublished data from the NCHS Master Facility Census; U.S. Bureau of the Census, *Preliminary Estimates of the Population of the United States, by Age and Sex: April 1, 1960 to July 1, 1971,* Series P-25, No. 483, April 1972; U.S. Bureau of the Census, *Estimates of the Population of the United States, by Age, Sex, and Race: 1970 to 1975,* Series P-25, No. 614, 1975.

[a]For 1963-1969 this figure represents the sum of the NCHS Nursing Care Home and Personal Care Home with Nursing categories; and for 1971 and 1973 the figure represents the number of Nursing Care Homes.

[b]Figures are average annual rates of change from the year of the preceding column to the year for which the figure is shown.

[c]NA = Not Available.

The dominance of proprietary beds, a characteristic of nursing home provision in this country at least since the 1940s, increased somewhat over the study period—from 60 percent in 1963 to 68 percent of all licensed beds in 1973—after reaching a peak of 73 percent in 1971. That peak was matched by a corresponding drop in the proportion of beds under private, nonprofit auspices in 1971. Except for that dip, the number of private, nonprofit operated beds relative to all nursing home beds remained approximately the same—around 23 percent—in spite of a better than 100 percent increase in absolute number of these beds. The absolute number of government operated beds grew very little over the course of the study decade so that the percentage of total nursing home beds under government ownership dwindled from 16 percent to less than 10 percent.

The proportion of total facilities under proprietary ownership—though higher than the proportion of beds because proprietary homes have been on average much smaller than either private nonprofit or government facilities—fell from 82 percent in 1964 to 74 percent in 1973. This occurred, as we shall see, both because the average size of proprietary homes has increased much more than the average size of other nursing homes has increased, and because the smaller proprietary facilities of earlier years were the principal victims of facility closures. Although we cannot substantiate this conclusively with available data, it seems likely that the growth in nursing homes which took place over the study period resulted more from the construction of new facilities than from the expansion of older facilities. Developments in standards enforcement, as discussed in chapter 6, indicate that this must have been the case.

Many believe that nursing home use has become misuse. Reports of inappropriate institutionalization and pleas for the expansion of alternative means of providing long-term care abound. It is frequently argued that demand for nursing home beds follows supply and that as long as we continue to expand nursing home capacity, we will abort the development of alternatives. Thus, many policymakers and would-be policymakers inside of government and out have been advocating that controls be placed on further expansion of nursing home care provision. Inclusion of nursing homes under Public Law 93-641, the National Health Planning and Resources Development Act of 1974, reflects, in part, an outgrowth of that concern.

Perhaps an even more important source of increased governmental concern over nursing home care has been the dramatic rise in costs for such care, especially soaring government costs under Medicaid, the principal funding source for government sponsored nursing home care since the mid-1960s. The Medicare share of public nursing home costs, though significant at first, has shrunk from approximately 21 percent ($367.0 million) in 1968-1969 to around 5 percent ($255.0 million) of all federal nursing home payments ($5.3 billion) in 1976. It had shrunk to just 12 percent ($247.0 million) by 1971. For most of the study period, then (given that Medicare did not begin payments until 1967), the role of Medicare has been very small.[1]

Table 2-3 indicates expenditures, public and private, for each year, 1960 through 1976. The public share of these expenditures has grown from 21 to 53 percent. Moreover, 37 percent of all Medicaid spending in 1975 went for nursing home care.[2] According to the *National Journal*, nursing home payments as of November 1977 accounted for the bulk of Medicaid expenditures in nineteen states.[3] In some states, the percentage of nursing home residents whose care is paid for in some part by Medicaid runs as high as 75 percent.[4] National Medicaid expenditures on nursing home care totaled $5.0 billion in FY 1976.[5] Since it has been argued that many in nursing homes could be cared for at lower cost as well as more appropriately at home or in other less institutionalized supportive settings, considerable interest exists in locating the proper levers to use in molding the future shape of long-term care provision in this country.

Table 2-3
National Nursing Home Expenditures by Source of Funds, 1960-1976
(in millions)

	1960	1961	1962	1963	1964	1965	1966	1967	1968	1969	1970	1971	1972	1973	1974	1975	1976ᵃ
Public																	
Total	108	174	275	337	406	494	692	1,192	1,466	1,726	1,665	1,973	2,465	3,173	3,806	5,014	5,856
Federal	45	81	137	157	203	211	336	775	912	1,066	1,001	1,196	1,444	1,849	2,277	2,912	3,417
State & Local	62	94	138	180	203	283	356	418	554	660	664	777	1,022	1,323	1,524	2,097	2,439
Private																	
Total	419	432	420	554	809	830	835	666	604	735	1,195	1,309	3,395	3,477	3,649	4,086	4,744
Consumers	411	422	409	540	789	809	811	646	584	715	1,173	1,286	3,370	3,449	3,619	4,054	4,706
Other	8	10	11	14	20	21	24	20	20	20	22	23	25	28	30	32	38
Total	526	606	695	891	1,215	1,324	1,526	1,858	2,070	2,461	2,860	3,282	5,860	6,650	7,450	9,100	10,600

Source: *Social Security Bulletin*, "National Health Expenditures" issues: August 1964; January 1966; February 1967; April 1968; January 1969-1977.
ᵃPreliminary estimates.

Variations in Growth and Utilization

At the same time as the use of nursing homes has been on the rise nationally, growth of nursing home bed stocks and related rates of nursing home utilization have continued to vary greatly among states. Between 1967 and 1973, as shown from NCHS data in table 2-4, the bed stock of nursing homes and related facilities grew by less than 30 percent in sixteen states while they expanded more than 75 percent in five states. Nursing home bed supplies as of 1973 ranged from 2.2 per 100 elderly in West Virginia to 10.2 per 100 elderly in Wisconsin. Fourteen other states had more than seven nursing home beds per 100 elderly population while nine states in addition to West Virginia had fewer than four beds per 100 elderly.

Study Objectives

The study reported here was designed to assist in better understanding the demographic, economic, and programmatic reasons for the rapid growth in nursing home care over the period 1964-1974, and for the differences across localities in the utilization of nursing homes. The analysis was undertaken to enhance federal policymakers' understanding of the dynamics of the bed supply, and to provide state and local authorities with insights into the impact of their nursing home policies and programs.

Understanding the forces at work is important. As noted, differences in nursing home utilization levels when projected for the nation have significant budgetary implications as well as quality-of-life significance for a large number of impaired persons and their families who may seek nursing home care. In addition, if national nursing home policies continue to reflect the "medical model," utilization levels could hold important implications for medical manpower needs and supply and, consequently, for the cost of such manpower in other sectors of the health care system.

It seems particularly important that we understand the effects of governmental policies on nursing home growth and use levels, for unless such impacts are understood, it will be extremely difficult to predict the results of alternative policies and thus to select rationally from among them. If, for example, it appeared desirable at some point to fully finance nursing home care at the federal level with uniform reimbursement and regulatory policies, what levels of supply, utilization, and costs might be expected? Would states with low utilization levels experience increased utilization or would high use states experience declines in utilization levels?

As indicated, those seeking answers to such questions could be greatly assisted, it seems, by empirically derived knowledge of what has created growth and variation in utilization in the past. This calls for an understanding of the influence of not only the policies themselves but of other variables with which

Table 2-4
Growth Rates in Nursing Home Beds by State, 1967-1973

State	Number of Nursing Home Beds[a]			Number of Nursing Home Beds per 1,000 Population 65 and Over[a]		
	1967	1973	Percent Change 1967-1973	1967	1973	Percent Change 1967-1973
Alabama	8,806	14,075	59.8	29.2	39.4	34.9
Alaska	139	606	336.0	23.2	75.8	226.7
Arizona	3,988	6,430	60.8	31.0	32.8	5.8
Arkansas	10,478	17,338	65.5	47.2	67.2	42.4
California	85,105	149,031	75.1	51.7	77.3	49.5
Colorado	10,918	16,537	51.5	61.7	82.7	34.0
Connecticut	15,924	23,294	46.3	58.5	76.1	30.1
Delaware	1,492	2,213	54.9	34.9	47.1	35.0
District of Columbia	2,071	3,147	52.0	30.0	44.3	47.7
Florida	22,139	34,956	57.9	28.9	29.4	1.7
Georgia	11,236	25,859	130.1	33.2	64.3	93.7
Hawaii	1,327	2,726	105.4	34.0	53.5	57.4
Idaho	2,978	4,190	40.7	46.5	56.6	21.7
Illinois	49,478	75,019	51.6	46.7	66.7	42.8
Indiana	21,929	31,480	43.6	46.3	61.4	32.6
Iowa	27,998	32,409	15.8	81.4	90.8	11.5
Kansas	17,372	21,239	22.3	67.3	76.7	14.0
Kentucky	11,841	17,922	51.4	36.5	50.5	38.4
Louisiana	10,313	14,659	42.1	36.6	44.6	21.9
Maine	5,704	8,092	41.9	49.6	66.9	34.9
Maryland	10,409	16,965	63.0	39.0	52.0	33.3
Massachusetts	38,604	50,367	30.5	62.7	77.3	23.3
Michigan	28,739	47,810	66.4	39.6	60.7	53.3
Minnesota	28,837	42,260	46.5	73.0	99.4	36.2
Mississippi	3,766	7,882	106.6	17.8	32.2	80.9
Missouri	22,860	32,924	44.0	42.6	56.5	32.6
Montana	3,170	4,638	46.3	47.3	65.3	38.1
Nebraska	11,560	16,042	38.8	65.3	84.9	30.0
Nevada	749	1,482	97.9	38.8	39.0	35.4
New Hampshire	4,021	5,713	42.1	52.2	68.0	30.3
New Jersey	22,888	34,430	50.4	35.1	46.9	33.6
New Mexico	1,964	2,991	52.3	30.7	36.5	18.9
New York	60,341	90,447	49.9	31.7	45.5	43.5
North Carolina	14,181	21,989	55.1	37.4	48.2	28.9
North Dakota	4,909	6,493	32.3	76.7	92.8	21.0
Ohio	48,059	63,772	32.7	50.1	61.5	22.8
Oklahoma	19,374	26,100	34.7	69.7	81.3	16.6
Oregon	13,518	17,052	26.1	64.7	69.6	7.6
Pennsylvania	47,331	65,127	37.6	38.7	49.2	27.1
Rhode Island	4,876	6,361	30.5	50.3	58.4	16.1
South Carolina	4,720	7,979	69.0	26.8	37.6	40.3
South Dakota	5,198	7,489	44.1	66.6	90.2	35.4
Tennessee	8,449	14,183	67.9	23.6	34.3	45.3
Texas	43,988	73,947	68.1	48.9	68.2	39.5
Utah	3,777	4,476	18.5	54.0	52.7	2.4
Vermont	2,682	3,812	42.1	57.1	76.2	33.5
Virginia	10,062	15,678	55.8	29.9	39.4	31.8
Washington	17,378	30,969	78.2	57.4	90.0	56.8

Table 2-4 continued

	Number of Nursing Home Beds[a]			Number of Nursing Home Beds per 1,000 Population 65 and Over[a]		
State	1967	1973	Percent Change 1967-1973	1967	1973	Percent Change 1967-1973
West Virginia	2,186	4,563	108.7	11.5	22.4	94.8
Wisconsin	25,793	50,499	95.8	57.1	102.0	78.6
Wyoming	982	1,896	93.1	33.9	59.3	74.9
United States	836,554	1,277,458	52.7	44.5	59.9	34.6

Source: NCHS, *Health Resources Statistics, 1969,* and unpublished data from the 1973 NCHS Master Facility Census.

[a]Includes nursing care homes, personal care homes with and without nursing, and domiciliary care homes.

such policies may interact. For example, to what degree are differences in nursing home utilization levels across states attributable to differences in need for such care among the states' populations? Do some states have high use because they possess particularly large populations of older elderly—those over eighty or eighty-five—who are more likely to be functionally impaired than younger elderly?

Are there significant differences across locales in the availability of informal supports for these impaired individuals and hence in their propensity to seek nursing home care? The relative prevalence of married elderly, if variable, for example, could well affect level of demand for nursing home care across states. As Pollak has shown in table 2-5, marital status has a lot to do with the fact that nursing home utilization levels are higher for women than for men. The table shows that regardless of sex or age, nursing home admission rates are considerably lower for elderly who are married than for those who are not. Moreover, the table reveals that among unmarried elderly (who make up 89 percent of the nursing home population) in all age brackets, use rates are very similar for both sexes. From this, Pollak argues, it is clear that women dominate the nursing home population at all age levels in large part because they are so much more often unmarried.[6]

Close proximity of adult children to provide support for impaired parents would seem to be less common in states that have experienced large-scale outmigration. Thus, do differences in this factor account for some of the interstate variation in nursing home use?

Are some ethnic groups less prone to use nursing homes, relying instead upon three-generation households to care for infirm relatives? Substantial differences in ethnic composition of states' populations might then account for variations in level of nursing home utilization. The size of the black population may be particularly important.

Table 2-5

Utilization of Nursing Home Care within Age, Sex, and Marital-Status Groupings *(in percentages)*

Population Characteristics	Ages 65-74			Ages 75-84			85+	Total 65+
	Total	65-69	70-74	Total	75-79	80-84		
1. Total population	1.4	1.0	2.0	6.0	4.2	9.1	16.6	4.0
2. Married	0.3			1.8			5.4	0.8
3. Not married	3.0			8.8			19.7	7.1
4. Male	1.2	1.0	1.6	4.2	3.1	6.3	11.7	2.8
5. Female	1.6	1.0	2.2	7.2	5.0	10.8	19.4	4.8
6. Male—married	0.3			1.4			4.6	0.8
7. Male—not married	4.3			9.2			16.8	7.7
8. Female—married	0.4			2.4			7.1	1.0
9. Female—not married	2.5			8.7			20.8	6.9

Source: William Pollak, "Utilization of Alternative Care Settings by the Elderly," in M. Powell Lawton et al., eds., *Community Planning for an Aging Society* (Stroudsburg, Pa.: Dowden, Hutchinson and Ross, Inc., 1976), Table 5, p. 120. Reprinted with permission.

Census data indicate that 2.3 percent of black women and 1.9 percent of black men over sixty-five years of age reside in nursing homes. For whites the percentages are 5.1 and 2.9, respectively. As Pollak has observed, these rather striking differences between the use rate of blacks and whites exist in spite of the fact that the black aged, on average, have lower incomes and, as shown in table 2-6, greater disabilities—both factors that would appear to predispose individuals to nursing home use—than do the white elderly.

In seeking to explain this conundrum, Pollak initially hypothesized that use levels for blacks were lower due to this regional concentration in the southeastern states, which tend to have low utilization levels. In table 2-7, however, Pollak shows that nursing home use levels are lower for blacks in every state with a black aged population of at least 5,000 except Massachusetts. On the basis of these data, Pollak concluded that whatever factor(s) is keeping the nursing home use rates of blacks below those of whites is operating nationwide.[7]

Table 2-6

Differentials in Health Characteristics of the Aged by Color

	Limitations of Activity (%)	Number of Bed-Disability Days per Person per Year	Number of Restricted-Activity Days per Person per Year
White	45.3	11.8	33.9
Nonwhite	54.3	18.6	41.9

Source: William Pollak, "Utilization of Alternative Care Settings by the Elderly," in M. Powell Lawton et al., eds., *Community Planning for an Aging Society* (Stroudsburg, Pa.: Dowden, Hutchinson and Ross, Inc., 1976), Table 6, p. 121. Reprinted with permission.

Table 2-7
Nursing Home Utilization Rates by Race and State, 1970

State	White Nursing Home Population as a Percentage of Total Population over 65	Black Nursing Home Population as a Percentage of Total Population over 65
Alabama	3.72	0.73
Alaska	5.42	0
Arizona	1.82	2.49
Arkansas	4.47	2.49
California	4.85	3.13
Colorado	5.30	2.19
Connecticut	4.83	3.29
Delaware	3.41	0.51
District of Columbia	7.09	2.07
Florida	1.99	1.36
Georgia	3.99	1.25
Hawaii	0.25	0
Idaho	4.68	5.74
Illinois	4.35	2.29
Indiana	4.09	3.19
Iowa	6.39	6.92
Kansas	5.99	2.80
Kentucky	3.35	2.80
Louisiana	4.22	1.54
Maine	3.72	2.25
Maryland	3.66	2.36
Massachusetts	5.67	6.48
Michigan	4.16	2.97
Minnesota	7.19	7.43
Mississippi	2.60	0.22
Missouri	3.88	1.67
Montana	4.85	6.52
Nebraska	6.35	3.43
Nevada	2.35	0.57
New Hampshire	4.90	5.63
New Jersey	2.92	2.30
New Mexico	2.14	3.21
New York	3.16	1.74
North Carolina	3.02	1.47
North Dakota	7.50	22.72
Ohio	4.31	3.01
Oklahoma	5.82	3.82
Oregon	4.99	3.51
Pennsylvania	3.42	1.71
Rhode Island	4.08	5.04
South Carolina	3.25	1.32
South Dakota	6.69	0
Tennessee	2.23	1.18
Texas	5.04	2.37
Utah	3.48	0
Vermont	4.52	0
Virginia	3.08	1.84
Washington	5.67	3.26
West Virginia	1.64	1.31

Table 2-7 continued

State	White Nursing Home Population as a Percentage of Total Population over 65	Black Nursing Home Population as a Percentage of Total Population over 65
Wisconsin	5.56	5.70
Wyoming	3.94	10.34

Source: William Pollak, "Utilization of Alternative Care Settings by the Elderly," in M. Powell Lawton et al., eds., *Community Planning for an Aging Society* (Stroudsburg, Pa.: Dowden, Hutchinson and Ross, Inc., 1976), Table 8, p. 122. Reprinted with permission.

There is some reason to believe that the income level of a state's population may play some role in that population's propensity to use nursing homes. Both health and capacity to pay for home care or other care modes not covered by public subsidy tend to be inversely related to income. Do some states have low levels of nursing home utilization, therefore, because they have large poor populations?

Is high utilization in some states explained by their high level of urbanization? Nursing homes are likely to be more accessible because there are more of them in closer proximity to significant segments of the population in metropolitan areas. On the other hand, alternatives to nursing homes, especially greater availability of home care services, are also more plentiful in urban locations so that there may be less reliance on nursing homes for care of the impaired. Nonetheless, does the life-style of an urbanized population still mean that it will make greater demands for nursing home care?

What is the effect of climate on variability in levels of nursing home use? The highest rates do occur in the north central region of the country, where winters are the most harsh. Is there a causal connection? It is obvious that a harsher climate makes independent living for an impaired person more difficult. Perhaps climate becomes most critical where population densities are low and where supportive services may be a considerable distance away.

Given level of need and propensity among the population to utilize nursing homes, the relative access to such care could play an important role in explaining variations across states in utilization levels. Here state policies may be crucial.

States with low nursing home use may rely to a greater degree on other modes of caring for their elderly populations. Are mental hospitals used more extensively in these states? Is there greater availability of home care services or supportive residential environments—for example, personal care homes? If so, such availability may reflect state funding policy by which greater resources are put into these alternative care modes or, alternatively, in which the state underfunds nursing home care so that cheaper care settings must be used by the impaired population who in other states would enter nursing homes.

Is nursing home use in some states greater because eligibility criteria in those states are or have been more liberal, or because they include the medically needy, not just public assistance recipients under their medical assistance programs? Do some states have lower levels of nursing home use because they are more restrictive in their screening for medical need?

To what extent do differences across states in nursing home use reflect state policies that presumably determine supply of nursing home beds? Has high growth occurred in some states because reimbursement rates have been raised substantially or because those states altered their methods of rate determination—for example, from facility independent to reasonable cost? Have other states experienced slow growth of the nursing home bed supply because capital investment subsidization has been limited or because the health department responsible for issuing operating licenses to nursing home operators has imposed a restrictive certificate-of-need policy? Or has rigorous standards enforcement discouraged investors or resulted in the closing of many older facilities?

While we cannot hope to provide conclusive answers to all of these questions, it is to the search for answers to questions such as these that the remainder of this book is devoted. The central concern is to learn what determines growth in nursing home bed supply and utilization. To cast light on that question, it will be necessary at times to focus on explaining differences across states in utilization levels at a particular point in time—for example, 1964 or 1969. Some of those factors identified as important in explaining differences in utilization levels, of course, will be found to exert a negative impact on growth, while others will be found to enhance the prospect of growth. Before addressing these questions directly, we turn in the next chapter to a description of the study method employed in our quest for answers.

Notes

1. See "Long-Term Care—The Problem That Won't Go Away," *National Journal*, November 5, 1977, p. 1727; and Robert A. Heil, "Nursing Home Costs Are Rising—And So Is Government Share," *Modern Nursing Home*, May 1973, pp. 48-51.

2. Marjorie Smith Mueller and Robert M. Gibson, "National Health Expenditures; Fiscal Year 1975," *Social Security Bulletin*, February 1975, pp. 7-9.

3. "Long-Term Care—The Problem That Won't Go Away," p. 1727.

4. Data collected through site visits to ten states and a phone survey of forty-four states carried out by The Urban Institute in 1976 and 1977.

5. "Long-Term Care—The Problem That Won't Go Away," p. 1727.

6. William Pollak, "Utilization of Alternative Care Settings by the Elderly" in M. Powell Lawton et al., eds., *Community Planning for an Aging Society* (Stroudsburg, Pa.: Dowden, Hutchinson and Ross, Inc., 1976), pp. 120-121.

7. Pollak, p. 123.

Study Method

As indicated in chapter 1, the study reported was carried out as part of The Urban Institute's Nursing Home Supply and Demand Study, and consists of case study analyses of nursing home supply and demand in ten states. In addition, correlations for a number of sociodemographic variables were computed to assist in the case study analysis, and information on a number of key program variables was collected by telephone survey from various officials in thirty-four additional states. In this chapter we describe the study methods employed, beginning with an overview of the state sample selection process and concluding with a comparison between the nursing home bed growth pattern in the sample and that of the nation as a whole. A detailed description of the method employed in selecting the sample states is presented in appendix E.

Selection of a Representative Sample

The principal objective of the study reported here was to gain an understanding of the dynamics of the increasing supply and utilization of nursing home care. We were not seeking necessarily to maximize the amount of national growth over the period 1964-1974 that we could account for. Had that been the objective, we would have chosen those ten states with the largest bed supplies. Seeking to include a combination of states that account for a significant portion of the national nursing home population so that the generalizability of findings would be enhanced was one consideration in the selection of the states, however. It may be noted that the final sample of states does account for 31 percent of the country's nursing home population (see appendix E).

Since we desired an understanding of the dynamics and subtleties of nursing home expansion, we sought a sample of states with diverse experience. It was first of all essential to work with a group of states that represented a wide range of rates in nursing home growth. Thus, the primary selection criterion was the rate at which nursing home utilization (number of nursing home residents per 100 elderly population) increased over the study period, 1964-1974. Using this criterion, all fifty states were divided into quintiles. From this it was decided to choose states from the first, third, and fifth quintiles. Other selection criteria were then applied to insure diversity in state characteristics known or hypothesized to influence the level of nursing home growth (see appendix E).

Upon selection of the twelve states, officials of various state agencies and nursing home associations with policy responsibilities directly affecting nursing homes were contacted to learn the status of data availability and their willingness to participate in the study. State officials contacted included those in licensure, welfare, Medicaid, Hill-Burton, and health planning agencies as well as executive directors of state nursing home associations. Upon completing a telephone survey of these officials, Arizona was dropped for lack of data and replaced with another retirement state, Florida. Key officials in Minnesota expressed interest in the study but decided that time constraints would not permit them to participate. Minnesota was therefore replaced by Wisconsin, the state most similar to Minnesota. Texas and Virginia were later dropped from the sample as explained below. The final sample of states, then, consisted of Alabama, California, Florida, Mississippi, New Jersey, New York, South Dakota, Vermont, West Virginia, and Wisconsin.

Site Visits

Site visits of up to one week were made over a period of eleven months to each of the sample states. During these visits, state data on the number of nursing home beds and facilities by licensure category as well as reimbursement rates, occupancy rates, and number of licensed domiciliary care home beds were gathered where available. The vast bulk of effort going into site visits was spent interviewing state officials (and sometimes local officials) responsible at some point during the study period for making or implementing policies directly affecting nursing homes. The number of respondents varied from state to state, but officials interviewed in each state included those in licensure, welfare, Medicaid, Hill-Burton, and planning agencies as well as spokesmen for one or more of the associations of nursing home providers.

State Analyses

From data collected and from information and perceptions recorded in these interviews, we attempted to piece together for each state the explanation for that state's nursing home bed growth pattern experienced over the course of the study decade. The purpose of these state analyses was to see if a pattern of explanation for growth emerged across the different locales and also to gain insight into the role of state policies in shaping growth.

Approximately two-thirds of the way through the planned site visits and state analyses, it was decided to drop Texas and Virginia from the sample. After having analyzed growth in Alabama, West Virginia, and Mississippi, it became apparent that a rather common pattern of growth had occurred among southern states and that it was no longer advantageous to oversample that region. We did wish, however, to retain Florida in the sample because of its unique status as the foremost retirement state.

The decision to proceed with the analysis without replacing Texas and Virginia in the sample was based on several considerations. We became convinced that new insights to be gained would be minimal and that, consequently, resources would be better utilized by a more thorough analysis of the ten-state sample, including the compilation and analysis of sociodemographic data on those states from the 1960 and 1970 Censuses.

In addition, the selection of two replacement states was complicated by the fact that we could not insure that the states selected would be representative in terms of growth and utilization level of those states not already heavily represented in the ten-state sample. The discrepancies between the NCHS bed counts—the only data available with which to select a sample of states—and the actual number of beds licensed by the state in each of the study years, though in the same ball park, precluded such precision. For example, NCHS data covering the study decade indicate that Mississippi was a low initial utilization, moderate growth state while both California and South Dakota were states with moderate initial utilization and high growth. As it turns out, using state licensure agency bed counts, Mississippi experienced high rather than moderate growth, California had a low rather than a moderate initial bed stock level, and South Dakota, rather than possessing a moderate-sized bed stock level at the outset of the study period, actually had a very high bed stock at that point. As these examples suggest, the NCHS counts are biased in both directions depending on the state, thus making it impossible to select precisely states with the desired bed growth and initial bed stock characteristics which would best "fill out" the sample. (See appendix C for a comparison of NCHS and state licensure data in the ten sample states.)

Telephone Survey

A telephone survey of various state officials concerned with nursing home policies in thirty-four additional states, carried out as part of the Nursing Home Supply and Demand Study, was also relied upon at points to enhance our ability to generalize from data obtained in the ten sample states. The six states excluded are those with the smallest populations. Information was obtained for a number of programmatic variables: reimbursement policies; proportion of nursing home residents supported by Medicaid and/or other public assistance; eligibility criteria, both financial and medical assessment; Life Safety Code enforcement and staffing requirements; certificate of need; supply of personal care homes; and capital funding subsidies.

Treatment of Data

The particular time span, 1964-1974, selected by HEW as the study period for investigation, is somewhat arbitrary, so that it will be extremely helpful at times to recount as best we can determine it the nursing home situation prior to the study period. Also, at some points in the analysis that follows, number of beds comprises the dependent variable while at other points the analysis relies on resident data. Although such a distinction at times is theoretically useful, the selection of one index over the other was necessitated at some points by data availability constraints. While these two indexes clearly are not one and the same, interchangeable use of them does not appear to create a major analytic problem because of the high occupancy rates that have characterized nursing homes.

Much of the picture of nursing home utilization and supply dynamics that emerges in the remainder of this book, especially that involving the impact of program variables, is based on insights obtained from the case studies and, to some degree, from findings of the phone survey of officials in thirty-four additional states.

In order to avoid confusion as to which statements in this report apply to the sample of ten states and which are projected to the universe of all fifty states, an uppercase form of the word "State" will be used from hereon whenever just the sample States are meant. Whenever the lowercase form is used, then, the reader may infer that both the sample and the universe, in general, are meant.

Growth among the Sample States

The ten sample States included in this study together experienced a 119 percent growth in number of nursing home beds during the period 1964-1974 (see table 3-1). The increase in number of beds per 100 elderly was 73 percent. The average annual percentage increase in number of beds in the ten States together measured 5.6 percent. Dividing the span of eleven years under study into three periods, we find that the average annual percentage growth in number of beds per 100 elderly in the years 1964 through 1966 averaged 8.3 percent; in the years 1967 through 1969, 7.2 percent; and over the period 1970 through 1974, 2.5 percent.

Thus, although the data are not directly comparable,[a] it appears that growth

---

[a]Determination of national growth is based on data from the National Center for Health Statistics' Master Facility Inventory censuses collected in 1967, 1969, 1971, and 1973; the growth pattern of the sample is based on State licensure data for each of the study years, although for some years the figures had to be estimated.

among the sample States was roughly similar to the growth rate nationally at the beginning, somewhat faster during the middle part of the period—right after the Medicaid and Medicare programs were enacted—and significantly slower during the early 1970s. It is apparent that the growth which did occur among the sample States during the middle part of study period—growth that many have attributed to the enactment of Medicare and Medicaid—was a continuation of a pattern of very rapid growth which preceded the adoption of these funding mechanisms. The much slower growth among the sample States during the final segment of the period seems too large to be accounted for by differences in the data. Part of the difference may be accounted for by the fact that California, which possesses 11 percent of the national nursing home stock, experienced a decline in growth during that time; and its pattern, obviously, had a much larger impact on the aggregate pattern of the sample States than it did on the national pattern. Likewise, since California experienced a very rapid growth in the mid-1960s, its presence in the sample may also account in part for the faster growth recorded among the sample States than for the country as a whole during the second segment of the period.

As depicted in table 3-2, our sample turned out to contain four States with "high" growth rates—Alabama, California, Mississippi, and South Dakota—two States with "high moderate" growth rates—Wisconsin and New Jersey—two States with "low moderate" growth—New York and West Virginia—and two States with "very slow" expansion—Florida and Vermont. Of those six States with high or high moderate growth, only Wisconsin and South Dakota began the period with high utilization levels. Initial bed stock levels in the other States, except New Jersey, were among the lowest. Two States with moderate growth, New Jersey and New York, also began the period with moderate-sized bed stocks. Of the two States with slow expansion, Vermont began the period with a large bed supply while Florida began with a relatively small bed stock. On the basis of this as well as compilations presented in table 3-1, we can see that there exists a moderate inverse relationship between initial utilization level and growth rate over the succeeding decade. That is, there was a tendency of those States with small bed stocks at the beginning to "make up" for this over the study period by expanding their bed stocks more rapidly.

It is of interest to note that two out of the four southern States included in the study—Alabama and Mississippi—fall into the group of high growth States. Moreover, both of these States had very small bed stocks at the outset of the study period. At the end of the period, Mississippi continued to experience rapid growth, the most rapid of any sample State at that point. Also, both of the north central States in the sample experienced either high or high moderate growth. In contrast to the southern States sampled, growth in these two States—Wisconsin and South Dakota—was relatively rapid in spite of an already

Table 3-1
Bed Supply: Ten-State Sample, 1960-1974

	1960	1961	1962	1963	1964	1965
Alabama		3,391	4,083	5,026	6,258	7,793
California	16,819	18,735	22,264	27,829	36,351	43,573
Florida			9,553	10,975	13,468	14,983
Mississippi				2,600	2,625	2,650
New Jersey					13,802[b]	15,372[b]
New York[a]					50,000	52,000
South Dakota					3,000[b]	3,405
Vermont			1,747	1,892	1,925[b]	1,975[b]
West Virginia		1,355	1,643	1,498	1,532	1,582[b]
Wisconsin					21,509	26,191
Total						
Number					150,470	169,524
% Increase—Beds					—	12.7
Beds per 100 Aged					2.55	2.82
% Increases—Beds/100 Aged					—	10.6
65+ Pop. (in 1000s)					5,879	6,001
% Increases—65+ Pop.					—	2.1

[a]10,000 beds added to number of licensed nursing home beds for each year 1964-1968 to account for "residential" beds later classified as ICF beds.
[b]Estimate.

large existing bed stock in 1964. The two industrial northeastern States—New York and New Jersey—appear to have had fairly similar growth patterns except for the last year of the period, although no reliable data are available on New Jersey for those years prior to 1970. Vermont, a rural northeastern State, experienced a slower growth but began the period with a much larger bed stock than either New York or New Jersey.

Ranking the sample States in terms of average annual percentage increases in bed stock does ignore the very great differences in size of the initial bed stocks among the sample States. As a result, States such as Mississippi or West Virginia with very small initial stocks (base numbers) can register very high percentage increases with only relatively small increases in absolute number of beds. To standardize or to control for this factor, the States also were ranked according to the ratio of bed stock in 1974 to bed stock in 1964. Figure 3-1 depicts the growth rates of the sample States when computed in this fashion. There is some rearrangement of States, but the order overall remains quite similar.

1966	1967	1968	1969	1970	1971	1972	1973	1974
9,045	9,646	10,557	11,983	12,527	12,784	13,668	15,191	16,703
53,988	58,949	69,200	75,631	93,166	95,220	96,765	96,601	97,777
16,657	18,339	21,557	23,062	25,400	26,607	27,956	29,262	29,796
2,948	3,301	4,060	4,968	6,669	7,571	7,772	7,983	8,892
16,624[b]	18,186[b]	18,907[b]	19,856[b]	20,768[b]	22,066[b]	22,375[b]	25,354	25,688
54,566	54,756	57,151	61,593	63,747	66,998	73,454	82,007	88,017
4,201	4,324	5,322	5,554	5,999	6,263	6,367	6,802	6,774
2,067	2,079	2,023	2,117	1,989	2,217	2,362	3,018	3,090
1,634[b]	1,687[b]	1,742[b]	1,799[b]	1,861	2,151	2,427	2,569	3,170
29,095	31,422	33,377	35,514	37,630	39,930	41,531	43,122	49,506
190,825	202,689	222,996	242,077	269,756	281,807	294,677	311,909	329,413
12.6	6.2	10.0	8.6	11.4	4.5	4.6	5.8	5.6
3.11	3.24	3.48	3.72	3.99	4.03	4.13	4.29	4.41
10.3	4.2	7.4	6.9	7.3	1.0	2.5	3.9	2.8
6,119	6,248	6,393	6,514	6,759	6,979	7,123	7,276	7,457
2.0	2.1	2.3	1.9	3.8	3.3	2.1	1.3	2.5

Before turning to the analysis of the impacts of governmental policies on nursing homes, it will be helpful to review in the next chapter certain very important sociodemographic and institutional developments that have impacted on the growth of nursing home care in this country.

Table 3-2
Initial Bed Stock Levels and Rates of Growth in Sample States,
1964-1974a

State	Initial Bed Stock Level	Average Annual Percent Increase in Bed Stock
California	1.8	10.7
Mississippi	1.3	9.7
Alabama	1.8	8.9
South Dakota	4.4	8.1
Wisconsin	5.0	6.4
New Jersey	2.2	5.5
New York	2.7	4.7
West Virginia	0.8	4.2
Florida	1.7	3.9
Vermont	4.3	3.4

aData availability considerations in the states dictated that the end points of
analysis be 1963-1973, 1963-1974, 1964-1973, or 1964-1974.

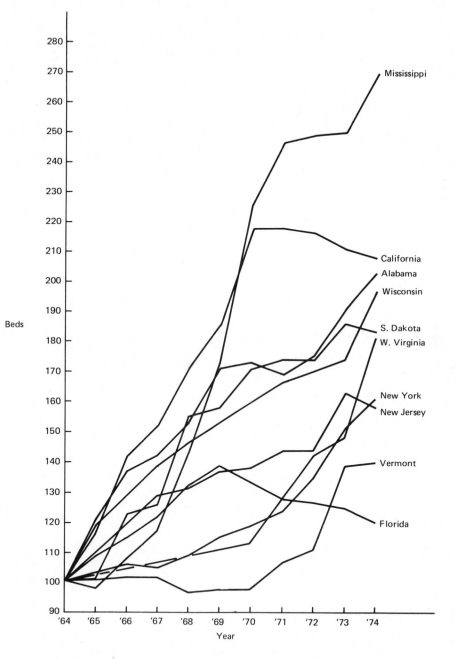

Figure 3-1. Ratio of Beds per 100 Elderly in Each Study Year to Beds per 100 Elderly in 1964 for 10 Sample States

4

Sociodemographic and Institutional Developments

In this chapter we take a look at some of the more clearly discernible changes that have occurred in the sociodemographic characteristics of the American population and in the preferred mode of caring for the nation's impaired elderly population—changes which help explain the major growth in nursing home use registered in this country over the period 1964-1974.

Sociodemographic Developments

As will become clear in later chapters, there is little doubt that governmental initiatives taken in the 1950s and 1960s to liberalize public subsidies for nursing home care greatly increased the effective demand for this service. Such actions, which became facilitators of nursing home use, however, were taken, at least in part, in response to a growing need perceived at both the federal and state levels for more nursing home beds. The recognition of the growing need for additional nursing home beds is evident in the work of the national Commission on Chronic Diseases in the early 1950s, in the record of congressional hearings (see, for example, "Hearing on H.R. 7341," House Committee on Interstate and Foreign Commerce, 83rd Congress, 2nd Session, 1954), and in various historical documents produced by health and welfare agencies in states such as California during that period. This need, in turn, clearly emanated from a series of important sociodemographic and economic changes that had taken place in this country, some of them with beginnings a number of decades earlier.[1]

Our treatment here of these changes will be brief—far more brief than such a complex subject deserves. A thorough analysis could easily comprise a substantial research effort in itself. Because most sociodemographic changes take place gradually, it is often impossible to measure these changes over a single decade. In addition, such developments occur in a very complex, contextual, and interactive fashion so that it is usually very difficult to isolate the impacts of discrete elements in these change processes. Nevertheless, a few of these changes have progressed with such swiftness in the last decade or two that their potential role in increasing demand for nursing home care over the years covered by this study cannot be ignored.

The most obvious of these factors is the aging of the elderly population. Between 1960 and 1970, according to census data, the elderly population (65 and over) nationally grew by 21 percent overall while numbers in the very oldest categories increased two and three times that rate (see table 4-1). Between 1965 and 1975, the segment of the elderly population between sixty-five and seventy-four rose 15 percent while that portion eighty-five and over increased 73 percent.[2]

This rapid growth in the size of the older elderly population is very significant because, as of 1960, 10 percent of the population eighty-five and over was residing in nursing homes—a rate of use nearly four times that of the youngest bracket of the elderly population. The reasons for this are quite obvious. On average, the level of impairment increases rather dramatically with age, especially after age seventy-five. Moreover, the chances of having a spouse or other family around to provide supportive care in case of impairment diminish significantly as age increases.

Using census counts, as indicated in table 4-1, of 388,000 elderly in nursing homes and related facilities in 1960, and 796,000 in 1970, Pollak has calculated that the change in age structure within the elderly population alone (assuming that utilization rates within each age bracket remained at 1960 levels) accounted for at least 14 percent of the increase in nursing home utilization nationally between 1960 and 1970.[3]

Utilization levels, however, as Pollak has pointed out, did not remain at their 1960 levels.[4] An increase in the rate of utilization of nursing home care has occurred within each age category of the elderly population. However, the increase has been much more dramatic at the upper end of the age bracket structure, where nursing home use was heaviest to begin with in 1960. This is evident in the figures of table 4-2, which show, for example, that between 1960 and 1970 nursing home utilization within the sixty-five to sixty-nine age bracket

Table 4-1
Population Aged 65 and Over by Age Groups: Totals and Percentages

	1960		1970			1980	
Population Group	*Number (1,000s)*	*Population 65+(%)*	*Number (1,000s)*	*Population 65+(%)*	*Increase 1960-1970(%)*	*Number (1,000s)*	*Population 65+(%)*
Total 65+	16,560	100	20,066	100	21	23,932	100
65 to 69	6,258	38	6,992	35	12	8,161	34
70 to 74	4,739	29	5,444	27	16	6,778	28
75 to 79	3,054	18	3,835	19	26	4,459	19
80 to 84	1,580	9	2,284	11	45	2,761	12
85+	929	6	1,511	8	63	1,773	7
65+ as a percentage of total U.S. population	9.2		9.3			10.1	

Source: William Pollak, "Utilization of Alternative Care Settings by the Elderly," in M. Powell Lawton et al., eds., *Community Planning for an Aging Society* (Stroudsburg, Pa.: Dowden, Hutchinson and Ross, Inc. 1976), Table 2, p. 117. Reprinted with permission.

Table 4-2
Breakdown of Population 65 and Over in Nursing Homes, 1960 and 1970

Age Group	1960			1970		
	Population in Nursing Homes (1960)[a]	Population (1960)[b]	Ratio: Nursing Home to Total Population	Population in Nursing Homes (1970)[c]	Population Total (1970)[d]	Ratio: Nursing Homes to Total Population
65+	388,000	16,560,000	0.023	796,000	20,066,000	0.040
65 to 69	40,000	6,258,000	0.006	70,000	6,992,000	0.010
70 to 74	66,000	4,739,000	0.014	107,000	5,444,000	0.020
75 to 79	89,000	3,054,000	0.029	164,000	3,835,000	0.043
80 to 84	95,000	1,580,000	0.060	207,000	2,284,000	0.091
85+	98,000	929,000	0.105	249,000	1,511,000	0.165

Source: William Pollak, "Utilization of Alternative Care Settings by the Elderly," in M. Powell Lawton et al., eds., *Community Planning for an Aging Society* (Stroudsburg, Pa.: Dowden, Hutchinson and Ross, Inc, 1976), Table 3, p. 117. Reprinted with permission.
[a]U.S. Bureau of the Census, *Census of Population: 1960, Final Report, Inmates of Institutions*, PC(2)-8A, Table 7.
[b]Ibid., *Census of Population: 1960*, Vol. I, *Characteristics of the Population*, p. 1-148.
[c]Ibid., *Census of Population: 1970, Persons in Institutions and Other Group Quarters*, PC(2)-E4, Table 6.
[d]Ibid., *Census of Population: 1970, General Population Characteristics, U.S. Summary*, PC(1)-B1, Table 52.

rose from 0.6 percent to 1.0 percent and that utilization by persons eighty-five and over grew dramatically from less than 11 percent to over 16 percent of the elderly in that age category. By the close of the study decade, a full 25 percent of the population eighty-five and over was residing in nursing homes.[5]

What then accounts for this significant increase in the rate of utilization of nursing homes, especially among the very old? Sociodemographic factors often referred to in the relevant literature as well as those variables frequently cited as explanations by our sample State respondents include increased population mobility, increased labor-force participation of women—the "traditional" source of most informal care, it is believed—and smaller houses unable to accommodate an extended-family member.

In an effort to assess quantitatively the impacts of some of these sociodemographic changes frequently offered as explanations for the expansion of nursing home use, correlations between changes in nursing home utilization level as measured in the census from 1960 to 1970, and changes from 1960 to 1970 in the values of several sociodemographic indexes contained in the census, were run for the forty-eight contiguous states. Indexes measured were percentage of elderly population seventy-five and over and eighty-five and over, percentage living with spouse, percentage of nonelderly female population employed in the labor force, percentage of elderly population residing in rural locales, percentage of elderly living dependently with children, percentage of elderly living alone, with nonrelatives, or in group quarters, and percentage of the elderly population that is black. Only three of these variables emerged with correlation coefficients of 0.25 or above: change in percentage of elderly population age eighty-five or over, 0.48; change in proportion of elderly living dependently, −0.28; and change in the percentage of nonelderly females participating in the labor force, 0.25.

In a multiple regression analysis (which allows one to measure the independent impact of a variable while holding the influence of other variables constant) carried out by the author several years ago, age structure, measured as the percentage of the elderly population that was seventy-five and over, emerged among nineteen independent variables as by far the most important factor in explaining the variation across States in nursing home utilization levels.[6] Similarly, in a recent extension of this kind of approach carried out by Scanlon, age structure, measured as percentage of elderly population eighty-five and over, again emerged as the principal explanatory variable.[7]

One variable not included in the correlations run on the forty-eight states, but one that has undergone measurable acceleration since 1940, is the level of geographic mobility or internal migration of the American population (see table 4-3). Such increased mobility would appear to make the availability of nearby relatives to care for an impaired family member less likely. Thus, taking some lag effect into account, this abrupt break with the slower rate characterizing the decades preceding 1940 may have created an appreciably greater need for

Table 4-3
Native Population by Residence Within or Outside State, Division, and Region of Birth, 1850-1970
(percent)

| | Born in State of Residence[a] | Born in Other States | | Born in Division of Residence | Born in Region of Residence |
		Contiguous to State of Residence	Noncontiguous to State of Residence		
1970[b]	67.9	9.3	17.4	75.1	79.4
1960[c]	70.3	9.8	16.5	77.8	82.0
1950[d]	73.5	10.4	14.8	81.1	85.4
1940	77.1	10.5	11.9	84.7	88.9
1930	76.2	11.2	12.1	84.2	88.8
1920	77.4	10.6	11.5	84.9	89.7
1910	78.0	10.1	11.4	85.1	90.3
1900	79.0	9.6	11.0	85.7	91.4
1890[e]	78.5	8.7	12.1	84.4	90.7
1880	77.9	9.4	12.7	84.1	90.9
1870	76.8	9.6	13.6	82.9	89.8

Source: Adapted from Table Series C 1-14, *Historical Statistics of the United States from Colonial Times to 1970*, U.S. Department of Commerce, 1975, p. 89.

[a]Prior to 1960, Alaska and Hawaii included in outlying areas.

[b]Based on 5 percent sample of persons enumerated.

[c]Based on 25 percent sample of persons enumerated.

[d]Based on 20 percent sample of persons enumerated.

[e]Excludes population of Indian territory and Indian reservations, specifically enumerated in 1890, with a native population of 117,368 white, and 208,083 Negro and other races, not distributed by state of birth.

nursing home care by the late 1950s and early 1960s, a point at which the rapid nursing home growth observed over the study period appears to have been already underway.

Other related developments less frequently offered as explanations may, in fact, also be significant and would seem to deserve future research attention. One is the increase in real family income that has taken place since 1960, better enabling the population to purchase nursing home care and, of course, alternatives such as home health care as well. Perhaps of more direct importance has been the substantially increased retirement incomes of the elderly through Social Security benefits and other pensions since the 1950s. (It appears unlikely that Social Security retirement benefits had much impact on the economic well-being of the elderly prior to the 1950s.)[8] Availability since that point, undoubtedly, has allowed more elderly to live alone. Their numbers increased from 18 to 26 percent of the elderly population between 1953 and 1970.[9]

Living-alone status, included among the correlations, has been found in any number of studies to be associated with likelihood of institutionalization. A causal connection has not been firmly demonstrated, however. The fact that elderly without family—the segment of the population with disproportionately high rates of nursing home admission—tend to live alone may account for much of the reported correlation between living-alone status and likelihood of nursing home admission. It is clear from available evidence that families, especially adult children, on the whole, continue to provide much emotional and social support to their elderly relatives and that most elderly individuals who have children live within a relatively short driving distance of at least one of them. Nonetheless, it may well be, as Manard and associates seem to suggest, that living-alone status does index, at least crudely, a level of household independence such that family members are less likely to be available to provide daily care support should the elderly relative living alone come to suffer serious impairment.[10]

It is also possible that the age cohorts reaching eighty or eighty-five over the past decade or two carry with them historically unique sociodemographic or cultural "baggage"—such as lower fertility rates which produced fewer children or siblings upon whom they can rely for support, or the financially devastating effects of the Depression—which manifested themselves in substantially reduced resources with which to protect themselves against the physical decrements of old age.

Again, detailed examination of the potential impacts of basic sociodemographic developments such as these on increased demand for and utilization of nursing home care in this country must be left to future analytic effort of a somewhat different focus. Their potential importance seems underscored by the observation that several other countries with similar demographic patterns but quite different programmatic arrangements appear to have experienced, on the whole, remarkably similar long-term care utilization levels and growth patterns.[11] Our consideration here of some of these developments, of course, remains largely suggestive rather than confirmatory.

Another source of increased nursing home utilization by the elderly in all age brackets is more clear-cut. That is the substitution of nursing home care for that formerly delivered in other settings. This transition in modal care setting is the development to which we next turn our attention.

Institutional Developments

It is evident that a substantial portion of increased nursing home utilization over the study period stems from the fact that nursing home care has come to replace much care that was formerly provided in other long-term care settings. Nursing homes in this country have become the central, long-term care setting for the nation's impaired elderly.

Table 4-4 presents data on the proportion of old persons in all types of

Table 4-4
Old People in Institutions, by Type of Institution, 1960 and 1970

	1960[a]		1970		Percentage Change, 1960-1970
	Number	Percent	Number	Percent	
Total number of people 65+	16,560,000[b]		20,066,000[c]		+21
Total 65+ in institutions	615,100	100	971,600[d]	100	+58
In nursing homes, personal care homes, and homes for the aged	388,000	63	795,800[e]	82	+105
In mental hospitals	177,800	29	113,000[f]	12	−36
In correctional institutions	800	—[g]	4,300[h]	—[g]	+432
In TB hospitals	14,200	—[g]	5,100[i]	—[g]	−64
In chronic-disease hospitals (other than TB)	23,200	8	35,200[i]	4	+52
In other institutions	11,000	—[g]	18,300[i]		+66

Source: William Pollak, "Utilization of Alternative Care Settings by the Elderly," in M. Powell Lawton et al., eds., *Community Planning for an Aging Society* (Stroudsburg, Pa.: Dowden, Hutchinson and Ross, Inc., 1976), Table 1, p. 114. Reprinted with permission.

[a]Figures for inmates of different institutions for 1960 are from U.S. Bureau of the Census, *Census of Population: 1960, Final Report, Inmates of Institutions*, PC(2)-8A, Tables 3-7.

[b]*Census of Population: 1960, op. cit.*, Vol. I, *Characteristics of the Population*, p. 1-148.

[c]*1970 Census of Population, General Population Characteristics, U.S. Summary*, PC(1)-B1, Table 52.

[d]*1970 Census of Population, Persons in Institutions and Other Group Quarters*, PC(2)-4E, Table 19.

[e]Ibid., Table 6.

[f]Ibid., Table 4.

[g]Less than 1 percent.

[h]*1970 Census of Population, Persons in Institutions and Other Group Quarters*, Table 3.

[i]Ibid., Table 26.

institutions in 1960 and 1970. The table reveals that the proportion of elderly in nursing homes increased by 69 percent, that the use of mental hospitals by the elderly actually declined by 48 percent, and that the use of all institutions by the elderly increased by 30 percent over the decade. Figure 4-1 demonstrates that within the group of all institutionalized elderly persons the percentage in nursing homes rose from 63 to 82 percent of all institutionalized elderly. Between 1960 and 1970 the proportion of elderly persons in nursing homes (including personal care homes and homes for the aged) increased 69 percent, from 2.34 to 3.96 persons per 100 elderly population.

Deinstitutionalization of Mental Hospitals

Care of the elderly in nursing homes has come to replace a substantial portion of care that was delivered formerly in mental hospitals. This substitution has taken

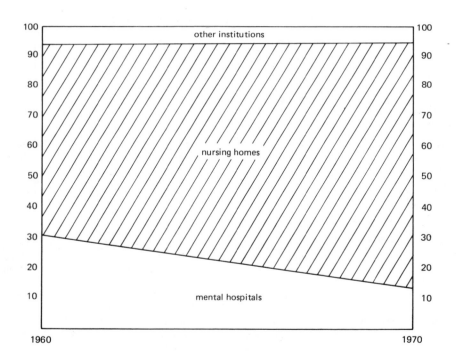

Source: William Pollak, "Utilization of Alternative Care Settings by the Elderly," in M. Powell Lawton et al., eds., *Community Planning for an Aging Society* (Stroudsburg, Pa.: Dowden, Hutchinson and Ross, Inc., 1976), Figure 3, p. 115. Reprinted with permission.

Figure 4-1. Percentage Distribution of Institutionalized Elderly by Type of Institution, 1960-1970

place for a number of reasons difficult to disentangle. The deinstitutionalization movement has been around for a number of years. Attention presently is focused on deinstitutionalization of the mentally retarded and other developmentally disabled. It began, however, with public mental institutions.

Deinstitutionalization can take one of two principal forms: the diverting to other settings at the intake or screening point of individuals who formerly would have been admitted to mental hospitals and, secondly, the placement of patients already in mental hospitals back into community settings. In most states, the former process appears to have preceded the latter. The Community Mental Health Center legislation passed during the early years of the Kennedy Administration comprised an initial impetus in some states and a further encouragement in others. Later court orders provided direct impetus in other states, particularly in the South.

There appear to be four principal explanations for the popularity of the deinstitutionalization concept. First was the idea that emerged among practitioners in the mental health field that care in a more natural or normal environment—that is, in the community—was more therapeutic than care in a large, depersonalized, geographically isolated institution. Undoubtedly, there were some advocating this position who were more concerned with the humaneness of such a treatment mode than they were with its therapeutic value, although these rationales soon became closely intertwined. Secondly, the use of psychotropic drugs made care in intensive environments less necessary for some individuals. Thirdly, it became "obvious" to many practitioners that a substantial number of elderly inmates did not really need to be in a mental institution but were placed there because there was no other setting in which they could be kept totally at public expense, and without the imposition on their families of a financial means test. Public mental hospitals had become a readily accessible means of caring for impaired old people, especially if they demonstrated any symptoms of senility.

These concerns of practitioners and reformers, which eventually became manifest in federal efforts to encourage states to make greater use of community mental health centers and other community alternatives, came to square very well with the fiscal interest of state executives and legislators. They soon came to see, especially with the passage of Medicaid and then the Supplemental Security Income Program (SSI) that if their patients were placed in privately operated community facilities rather than in the state and county mental hospitals, the federal government would pick up a substantial share of the care costs, which would be lower per diem than the costs of care in state hospitals anyway. In general, Old Age Assistance and then Medicaid discouraged the provision of care to persons in public institutions. Medicaid did permit reimbursement to public mental hospitals if they could qualify for accreditation from the Joint Commission on the Accreditation of Hospitals and if the state could demonstrate that it had plans underway to develop alternatives to use of state hospitals for the elderly.

With the confluence of all these forces, it is not difficult to understand the momentum that the deinstitutionalization movement acquired during the period of years covered by the study, 1964-1974. Census data reveal a 48 percent drop between 1960 and 1970 in the proportion of elderly residing in mental institutions (see table 4-4). Using these figures, Pollak has estimated that the diverting to nursing homes of elderly persons who formerly would have gone into mental hospitals could account for up to 32 percent of the growth in nursing home utilization between 1960 and 1970.[1,2]

The most consistent and reliable data on use of mental hospitals by state by year is available from the National Institute of Mental Health. Using that data for the sample States, as presented in table 4-5, we were unable to trace any particular growth spurt occurring in those States directly to state deinstitutionalization efforts. Rather, the impact presumably has been gradual as most of the sample States, like the nation as a whole, have experienced gradual declines in the proportion of their elderly populations residing in mental hospitals, at least since the mid-1960s. Some States—for example, California, New Jersey, New York, and Texas—began this gradual drop in use earlier than that. Heavy (though gradually diminishing) use of mental hospitals for the elderly throughout the study period in New York appears to explain some of the relatively low level of nursing home utilization there. Apparently New York was able to get more of its state mental hospitals certified for Medicaid reimbursement than other states were.

All of this indicates that the nursing home clearly was the primary long-term care setting by 1960, but that its dominance had increased immensely by 1970. A significant part of that increased dominance stemmed from increased substitution for care of the aged in mental institutions.

Specialization of Hospitals for Acute Care

Until relatively recently, hospitals were often used to care for impaired and usually indigent elderly on a long-term basis, especially if they required any amount of nursing care (see appendix A on the history of the nursing home). Some hospitals reserved special wings for long-term care, but this seems a largely post-World War II development. Use was especially heavy for public charges in county hospitals. By the beginning of the study period, however, specialization of hospitals for acute care (with all of its implications for facility prestige and rapidly rising costs) was nearly complete. This created increasing pressure to provide for the chronically ill or functionally impaired in specialized long-term care settings, principally nursing homes.

Data compiled on the number of long-term beds in general and chronic disease hospitals relative to the size of each sample State's elderly population indicate a steady decline in half of these States over the study period (see table

Table 4-5
Percent of Sample States' 65 and Over Population in Mental Hospitals, 1960-1975

State	1960	1961	1962	1963	1964	1965	1966	1967	1968	1969	1970	1971	1972	1973
Alabama	–	–	.64	.64	.64	.29	.70	.33	.63	.63	.56	.47	.35	.23
California	.83	.79	.74	.72	.62	.53	.43	.31	.23	.17	.11	.08	.05	.04
Florida	.40	.41	.41	.41	.40	.40	.39	.38	.33	.35	.14	.12	.11	.19
Mississippi	.59	.53	.57	.59	.61	.56	.60	.61	.60	.58	.53	.13	.50	.46
New Jersey	–	1.23	1.20	1.15	1.12	1.07	1.04	1.00	.92	.86	.75	.71	.64	.58
New York	1.74	1.71	1.68	1.65	1.64	1.67	1.63	1.61	1.58	1.45	1.34	1.23	1.11	.99
South Dakota	.90	.78	.78	.80	.85	.82	.73	.70	.62	.56	.51	.48	.43	.30
Texas	.57	.54	.52	.50	.47	.44	.25	.42	.40	.32	.28	.23	.19	.16
Vermont	.92	.99	1.05	1.02	1.01	.91	.86	.83	.71	.67	.83	.77	.66	.51
Virginia	1.06	1.04	1.01	1.00	1.00	1.03	1.03	1.08	–	.97	.90	.91	.64	.56
West Virginia	.70	.78	.66	.70	.69	.64	–	.64	.58	.71	.53	.45	.48	.43
Wisconsin	1.34	1.34	1.14	1.13	1.12	1.10	–	1.03	.87	.71	.60	.62	.46	.44

Source: National Institute of Mental Health, annual statistics published under varying titles; usually, "Patients in Mental Institutions: State and County Mental Hospitals," "Additions and Resident Patients at End of Year in State and County Mental Hospitals," and "Private Mental Hospitals and General Hospitals with Psychiatric Service." U.S. Department of Health, Education and Welfare.

4-6). In the remainder, a mixed picture prevails, and in two of those States, the numbers are too small to tell. In no State is there evidence of an *abrupt* change in the long-term hospital bed stock.

The 1965 enactment of Medicare made transfer from hospital to an extended care facility (ECF) for recuperative care financially feasible for many for the first time. By 1967 the Joint Commission on the Accreditation of Hospitals began requiring utilization review, at least on paper, as a condition of accreditation. Utilization review under Medicare (inaugurated with the establishment of the ECF program) and under Medicaid, as well as under private third-party insurers, has become progressively more stringent since that point, focusing upon emptying hospitals of long-term recuperative patients as well as the chronically ill. Enforcement of utilization review, however, may have been vigorous in only a small minority of hospitals during the study period.

Data on the mean length-of-stay in general hospitals, as displayed in table 4-7, reveal a mixed picture by sample State; but overall, they indicate a slight increase in average length of stay in the hospital. Perhaps the most obvious explanation for such an increase is that, with the introduction of Medicare, hospitals have gotten larger proportions of elderly. Although their hospital stays have been shortened from what they would have been prior to "utilization review," they undoubtedly stay significantly longer per hospital episode than the younger population who comprised the ranks of the hospitalized to a greater degree before Medicare was introduced. These data, however, are not really helpful for present purposes since there is no age breakout and thus not even an indirect way of separating out recuperative care from intense medical care.

Thus, although the available data do not provide a proxy measure of change in use of hospitals for the provision of recuperative and long-term care that can be traced directly to increased use of nursing homes for this purpose, it appears from several historical accounts that a significant substitution has developed over the past two or three decades and that this has contributed in some degree to the nursing home growth observed over the study period.[13]

Substitution for Care in Residential Group Settings

In addition to the increased use of nursing homes for much of the care formerly rendered in mental institutions and general hospitals, it seems likely—largely because of the greater availability of federal funding for nursing home care—that some substitution of the nursing home setting for supportive residential facilities (SRFs) has occurred as well. Again, clear-cut quantitative indicators are hard to come by. Such settings, which are meant to provide care above room and board but only limited, if any, nursing care, typically are licensed by states as "personal care homes," "sheltered care homes," "homes for the aged," and the like.

Table 4-6
Long-Term Care Beds in General and Long-Term Hospitals Per 100 Elderly in Sample States, 1960-1974

State	1960	1961	1962	1963	1964	1965	1966	1967	1968	1969	1970	1971	1972	1973	1974
Alabama	.04	.04	.04	.04	.04	.04	.03	.06	.03	0	0	0	0	0	0
California	.65	.63	.58	.69	.67	.66	.62	.57	.48	.40	.39	.35	.35	.34	.22
Florida	.01	.01	.01	.01	.01	.01	0	0	0	0	0	0	.02	.01	.01
Mississippi	.02	.02	.03	.03	.03	.03	.03	.03	.03	.03	.01	.01	.01	.01	.01
New Jersey	.53	.60	.64	.65	.78	.40	.41	.41	.57	.38	.36	.30	.18	.25	.27
New York	.85	.78	.77	.82	.63	.63	.49	.47	.49	.46	.42	.39	.41	.41	.36
South Dakota	.10	.09	.10	.09	.08	.08	.09	.09	.09	.09	.09	.09	.10	.10	.09
Texas	.08	.15	.16	.17	.14	.11	.11	.30	.26	.30	.28	.11	.06	.11	.10
Vermont	.06	.06	.06	.08	.08	.07	.07	.09	0	0	0	0	0	0	0
Virginia	.06	.05	.05	.05	.05	.05	.15	.24	.13	.13	.12	.09	.16	.15	.16
West Virginia	.10	.09	.09	.11	.12	.12	.31	.27	.20	.25	.24	.23	.25	.26	.25
Wisconsin	.32	.31	.39	.43	.35	.35	.35	.60	.29	.26	.24	.23	.25	.23	.25
Mean	.24	.24	.27	.27	.25	.21	.22	.26	.21	.17	.18	.15	.15	.16	.14

Source: American Hospital Association, Annual Guide issues of *Hospitals*, now called "Guide to the Health Care Field."

Table 4-7
Mean Length of Stay in General Hospitals in Sample States, 1960-1974

State	1960	1961	1962	1963	1964	1965	1966	1967	1968	1969	1970	1971	1972	1973	1974
Alabama	6.4	6.3	6.5	6.8	6.9	7.0	7.1	7.5	7.5	7.7	7.7	7.5	7.4	7.5	7.4
California	7.2	7.1	7.0	7.0	7.0	7.0	7.2	7.4	7.3	7.4	7.1	6.9	6.8	6.6	6.7
Florida	6.9	7.0	7.0	7.2	7.3	7.3	7.6	8.0	8.2	8.2	7.9	7.7	7.7	7.5	7.4
Mississippi	5.8	5.9	5.9	6.0	6.3	6.3	6.5	6.8	7.1	7.1	7.0	6.9	6.9	7.0	6.9
New Jersey	8.1	8.2	8.2	8.3	8.3	8.5	8.9	9.2	8.8	8.9	8.9	8.8	8.8	8.8	8.8
New York	9.7	9.7	9.7	9.7	10.0	9.9	10.1	10.6	10.4	10.5	10.4	9.8	9.6	9.8	9.8
South Dakota	7.0	6.8	6.9	6.8	7.0	7.0	7.1	7.6	8.0	7.9	7.9	7.3	7.2	7.3	7.3
Texas	6.0	6.1	6.2	6.4	6.5	6.6	6.7	7.0	7.3	7.3	7.2	7.1	7.1	7.0	6.8
Vermont	7.3	7.4	7.4	7.4	7.3	7.6	7.6	8.4	8.4	7.8	8.2	7.6	7.8	8.1	8.2
Virginia	7.7	7.7	7.7	7.8	7.9	7.9	8.0	8.4	8.5	8.3	8.4	8.4	8.1	8.2	8.1
West Virginia	7.1	7.4	7.3	7.3	7.4	7.5	7.5	7.8	8.0	8.0	8.1	7.9	7.9	7.7	7.7
Wisconsin	7.4	7.4	7.3	7.4	7.6	7.5	7.7	8.2	8.6	8.0	8.4	8.5	8.3	8.4	8.3
Mean	7.2	7.3	7.3	7.3	7.5	7.5	7.7	8.1	8.2	8.1	8.1	7.9	7.8	7.8	7.8

Source: American Hospital Association, Annual Guide issues of *Hospitals*, now called "Guide to the Health Care Field."

Of course, there is no way of isolating the portion of growth in nursing home care that reflects direct substitution for care that previously would have been provided in these supportive residential environments. Sketchy data on beds in all State-licensed personal care homes available in nine of the sample States suggest that an increase over the study period in personal care home beds per 100 elderly occurred in only two States, and that increase was small (see table 4-8). In fact, only four States—Alabama, Florida, New Jersey, and New York—showed a definite, absolute increase in number of personal care beds, irrespective of elderly population size. Four States experienced a drop in beds per 100 elderly, while in three States the bed stock level remained roughly the same. In none of the sample States were we able to identify through 1973 any wholesale or major reclassification of SRFs to nursing homes, or vice versa. Thus, growth patterns do not appear to be connected to this phenomenon. If such reclassification occurred, more than likely it took place after the Life Safety Code was made enforceable in Intermediate Care Facilities in 1974 (see chapter 6).

Nationwide data from the National Center for Health Statistics indicate that the number of beds in "personal care homes without nursing" and in "domiciliary care homes" increased about 32 percent, from 3.4 to 4.5 beds per 100 aged population over the period 1963 through 1971, the last year for which we have comparable data. Because the NCHS survey data are received directly from individual facilities, these figures undoubtedly reflect some unlicensed beds, however.

We have no way of identifying precisely the amount of growth in nursing home care attributable to the substitution of care that formerly was provided in unlicensed boarding homes, boarding houses, and the like. Using census data on number of persons residing in "group quarters," Manard and associates have shown that the proportion of elderly in all group settings who reside in "group quarters" has declined from 40.5 percent in 1940 to only 12.3 percent in 1970.[14] Moreover, the rate of decline accelerated over the course of the study period, dropping 42 percent since 1960. At the same time, the proportion residing in nursing homes increased from 34 to 72 percent between 1940 and 1970 (see table 4-9). Undoubtedly some of the drop in use of group quarters reflects substitution of nursing home care, but in actuality that portion may be quite small. Many who formerly ended up in boarding houses may with increased pensions now live alone in independent households rather than in other institutions. Another problem, of course, is that the census category of "group quarters" is ill-defined for our purposes, as it includes army barracks, college dormitories, and assorted other settings besides boarding homes and other "unlicensed" living arrangements used by the elderly.

Absence of reliable data on number of unlicensed boarding homes and the like from the sample States, unfortunately, prevents us from observing directly any relationship between growth in nursing home bed stock and use of boarding

Table 4-8
Supportive Residential Facility Beds per 100 Aged Population by Year in Ten Sample States, 1963-1974

State	1963	1964	1965	1966	1967	1968	1969	1970	1971	1972	1973	1974
Alabama	0.1	0.1	0.1	0.0	0.0	0.1	0.1	0.1	0.1	0.1	0.1	0.1
California	NA[a]	NA	NA	NA	NA	NA	NA	NA	NA	NA	NA	NA
Florida	0.21	0.36	0.32	0.56	0.57	0.68	1.08	0.89	0.94	1.24	1.32	0.31
Mississippi	NA	NA	NA	0.16	0.13	0.10	0.10	0.08	0.12	0.12	0.15	0.11
New Jersey	NA	NA	NA	0.3	0.4	0.6	0.8	0.9	1.0	1.2	1.4	1.5
New York	NA	NA	NA	NA	NA	NA	NA	NA	0.52	0.61	0.82	1.04
South Dakota	NA	NA	0.96	0.82	0.75	0.65	0.81	0.79	0.72	0.71	0.79	0.70
Vermont	1.5	NA	NA	1.2	1.3	1.2	1.2	NA	NA	NA	NA	NA
West Virginia	NA	NA	NA	NA	NA	NA	NA	NA	0.50	0.50	0.51	0.48
Wisconsin	NA	1.3	0.7	0.5	0.5	0.5	0.3	0.4	0.4	0.3	0.4	0.3

aNA = Not Available.

Table 4-9

Percentage Distribution of Institutionalized Elderly Population by Type of Institution, 1904-1970[a]

Type of Institution	1904[b]	1910	1940	1950	1960	1970
OAI			33.7[c]	35.2	49.7	72.4
Prison, reformatory	(2,851)[d]		0.8	0.5	0.4	0.2
Local jail or workhouse			0.5	0.4	0.3	0.2
Mental institutions	(20,374)[e]	(34,610)	23.5	22.9	23.2[f]	10.3
Tuberculosis hospitals				1.1	1.8	0.5
Other chronic disease hospitals				1.4	2.9	3.2
Homes and schools for the mentally handicapped	(34)			0.7	0.6	1.0
Almshouses	(52,795)	(46,032)				
Other institutions			0.9		2.8[g]	
Group quarters[h]			40.5	37.8	21.2	12.3
			100.0	100.0	102.9	100.1
Total population 65+ in institutions and group quarters	76,054	80,642	373,000	617,000	780,000	1,100,000

Source: Reprinted by permission of the publisher from *Old-Age Institutions* by Barbara Bolling Manard, Cary Steven Kart, Dirk W.L. van Gils (Lexington, Mass.: Lexington Books, D.C. Heath and Company, Copyright 1975, D.C. Heath and Company).

[a]1920 Census data does not distinguish persons living in institutions or group quarters from those living in single families. A "family" was defined as a group of persons, whether related by blood or not, who live together as one household. One person living alone is counted as a family; on the other hand, the occupants or inmates of a hotel or an institution are also counted as a single family.

1930 Census data distinguishes between families and "quasi-families." Quasi-families include institutions, boarding and lodging houses, hotels, schools, crews of vessels, labor camps, military and naval posts, etc. However, there is no information on the ages of persons living in quasi-families.

[b]These figures are based on "persons of known age" admitted during 1904 and does not correspond to the resident population of each institution. The age category for all 1904 figures is 60 years and over.

[c]The 1940 classification is "Homes for the Aged, Infirm and Needy" and includes almshouses, homes for the blind, the deaf, incurables, orphans, and disabled or aged soldiers and sailors.

[d]The 1904 Census does not include "reformatories."

[e]The 1904 classification is "Insane in Hospitals" and refers to hospitals caring only for the insane.

[f]The 1960 Census classification is "Mental Institutions and Residential Treatment Centers." Residential treatment centers were primarily intended to serve emotionally disturbed children. Contrary to expectation, however, the 1960 Census data shows that residential treatment centers often show more adult inmates than child inmates. Therefore, these are combined with mental institutions in one category.

[g]In 1960 "other institutions" represents a residual category of the difference between the total number of persons 65+ known to live in an institution and the total number of elderly persons known to live in specific types of institutions.

[h]"Group quarters" include persons living in boarding or lodging homes, labor camps, at military and naval posts, and so on.

homes at the individual state level. In an effort to pursue this further, however, the change in number of residents in group quarters between 1960 and 1970 was compiled from the census for each of the forty-eight contiguous states, and these data were then correlated with the change in bed growth for all these states. This exercise produced a correlation coefficient of −0.20, an indication that some substitution may have been taking place.

Formal Home Care

In addition to the substitution of nursing homes for care formerly rendered in other group settings—principally mental hospitals, general hospitals, and group residential settings—no doubt some proportion of nursing home growth reflects substitution for informal care formerly rendered in the home. In one State we were told that nursing home care also has come to replace some formal in-home care that used to be provided by public health nurses and physicians. It appears as well that the greater availability of private physicians who made house calls up to a decade or two ago, in conjunction with informal support provided by family, may have allowed a number of rather severely impaired and ill elderly to remain in their homes in the past.

Summary Observations on Institutional Developments

Surveying those long-term care modes that to a significant degree nursing home care has come to replace has allowed us to make at least three very important observations. First of all, growth in the level of institutionalization of the elderly in U.S. society appears to have been neither as extensive nor as rapid as may appear from a look at nursing home statistics or as many appear to have assumed. According to the very helpful analysis carried out by Manard and associates, the increase that occurred in the proportion of the elderly residing in group care settings of one type or another measured 140 percent between 1910 and 1970, an average annual increase of 2.3 percent.[15] The total numbers involved, however, are small—2 percent of the aged population in 1910 to 5.8 percent of that population in 1970. The difference indicated by those numbers probably is exaggerated because the base figure for 1910 reflects only those counted as residents of *institutions.* The number who were in "group quarters" in 1910, a category of residence included in the 1970 figures, is unknown for 1910. Instead of 2 percent in 1910, the true combined figure may well have been 3 percent. At any rate, the total percentage in 1940 was 4 percent, so that the 5.5 percent recorded for 1970, though very substantial, is not, it seems a staggering increase when spread over a thirty-year period.

Having said that, however, it is also necessary to point out that the growth in institutionalization of the elderly that has taken place in those thirty years since 1940 comprises one-half of all the increase that has occurred since the turn of the century (after an apparent dramatic increase from 1.5 to 2.8 percent of the aged population between 1890 and 1910).[16] This expansion was particularly rapid between 1940 and 1950, and then again between 1960 and 1970.

More significant for the present study is the growth since 1950 in the proportion of the total institutionalized elderly population who reside in nursing homes. This has been dramatic. Again, according to estimates developed by Manard and others, elderly in old age institutions (nursing homes plus personal care homes) comprised 35 percent of the total institutionalized population in 1950; but by 1970, that proportion had doubled to 72 percent.

What emerges from all this is a picture of relatively recent and very dramatic growth in the specialization of nursing homes for care that formerly was rendered in a number of institutionalized and residential settings. The nursing home has become the principal setting for the rendering of formal care to impaired elderly, especially those lacking family or financial resources. The reason for this development is quite clear. Nursing homes are where the federal government through OAA, MAA, and, most recently, Medicaid and Medicare, has put its matching health care dollars for providing long-term care.

In the next few chapters, we turn to a detailed discussion of additional explanatory factors investigated in this study. This discussion will show in some detail the specific routes through which the increased use of nursing home care for impaired elderly in U.S. society has come.

Notes

1. For a discussion of these developments, see J. Christopher Crocker, "A Brief History of Old Age Institutions in the United States," mimeographed (Charlottesville, Va.: University of Virginia, Center for Program Effectiveness Studies, 1974); and David Hackett Fischer, *Growing Old in America* (New York: Oxford University Press, 1977).

2. *Actuarial Study, No. 74.* Office of the Actuary, Social Security Administration, June 1974.

3. William Pollak, "Utilization of Alternative Care Settings by the Elderly" in M. Powell Lawton et al., eds. , *Community Planning for an Aging Society* (Stroudsburg, Pa.: Dowden, Hutchinson and Ross, Inc., 1976), p. 115.

4. Pollak, p. 115.

5. Arora Zappolo, "Characteristics, Social Contacts and Activities of Nursing Home Residents: United States: 1973-74, National Nursing Home Survey," *Vital and Health Statistics*, Series 13, No. 27, U.S. Department of Health, Education and Welfare, 1977.

6. See Burton Dunlop, "Determinants of Long-Term Care Facility Utiliza-

tion by the Elderly: An Empirical Analysis," Working Paper 963-35 (Washington, D.C.: The Urban Institute, 1973).

7. William Scanlon, "A Theory of the Nursing Home Market," Working Paper 5907-1A (Washington, D.C.: The Urban Institute, 1978).

8. See Crocker, p. 40.

9. See Barbara Manard et al., *Old Age Institutions* (Lexington, Mass.: Lexington Books, D.C. Heath and Company, 1975), p. 21; and David Hackett Fischer, p. 146.

10. Manard, p. 112.

11. See Ethel Shanas and Marvin Sussman, eds., *Family, Bureaucracy, and the Elderly* (Durham, N.C.: Duke University Press, 1977).

12. Pollak, p. 28.

13. The discussion in this section is drawn in large measure from the historical analyses contained in the following works: Robert Moroney and Norman Kurtz, "The Evolution of Long-Term Care Institutions," in S. Sherwood, ed., *Long-Term Care: A Handbook for Researchers, Planners and Providers* (New York: Spectrum Publications, 1975); William C. Thomas, Jr., *Nursing Homes and Public Policy* (Ithaca: Cornell University Press, 1969); R. Markus, "Nursing Homes and the Congress," Congressional Research Service, Library of Congress, November 1, 1972; "The Availability and Financing of Nursing Home Care," Blue Cross Reports: II, No. 2, April-June 1964; Helen McGuire, "New Laws and Regulations Must Focus on Continuity of Care," *Hospitals*, October 16, 1975, pp. 63-67; Manard; and Crocker.

14. Manard, p. 126.

15. Based on census data compiled by Manard, p. 129.

16. From census data reported by Crocker, p. 25.

Public Subsidization of Nursing Home Care

In this chapter we look at the methods through which federal and state governments subsidized demand for and supply of nursing home care over the period 1964-1974. Specifically, we analyze eligibility, reimbursement, and capital subsidy policies for their possible impacts on nursing home growth. This analysis will provide considerable insight into the means by which nursing homes have come to occupy the very dominant position they hold in the provision of long-term care today. Since the discussion presented here focuses on impacts at the state level, the reader may find it helpful before completing this section to review appendix B, which provides detailed discussions of subsidy policies as enunciated at the federal level.

Eligibility for Nursing Home Care

In the discussion of eligibility in this section, we will be concerned principally with formal eligibility criteria as enunciated at the state level. The interpretation and application of such statewide policies at the local level undoubtedly were subject to considerable variation even during the study period. However, a proper understanding of the potential impacts of such variations very likely would consume the entire resources of a study such as the one reported here—a study designed to determine the overall impacts of a number of variables, including eligibility policy, on nursing home bed growth.

As we learned in the interview phase of this study, very few respondents at the state level possessed knowledge of variations in policy applications that occurred at the local level or of the impacts of local policies. In some states, it was necessary to seek out respondents specifically knowledgeable about local procedures; but even then, such persons were typically familiar with only one or two localities. The one facet of eligibility procedures at the local level which State respondents seemed most confident about was that regarding the enforcement of a relative responsibility provision. "Relative responsibility" is the term applied in the welfare lexicon to provision of welfare statutes and regulations which require that close relatives, principally adult children, if capable, pay a portion of an elderly welfare recipient's income. It seems likely that many of the local governments that were contributing to the reimbursement costs for nursing home care tended to interpret state eligibility policy somewhat restrictively.

Finally, by way of preface, the discussion in this section will be concerned primarily with eligibility policy under medical assistance programs which preceded Medicaid—that is, Old Age Assistance (OAA), Assistance to the Aged, Blind and Disabled (AABD), and Medical Assistance for the Aged (MAA). A discussion of eligibility policy under Medicaid and Medicare will be deferred until the section which treats specifically the impacts of those programs on the growth and shape of the country's nursing home bed stock. However, it should be noted here that, in most states, eligibility policies under Medicaid, the successor to these earlier medical assistance programs, remained identical or quite similar to those in effect under earlier programs.

Program eligibility determination typically involves the application of three basic criteria: income level, assets level, and degree of relative responsibility. In the eligibility determination process for medical assistance, including nursing home care, a fourth criterion is applied; assessment of medical need for care. Among the financial criteria, income policy appears to be the most crucial, as it constitutes the principal determinant of the scope of any assistance program.

The key distinction with regard to impact of income eligibility determination on access to nursing home care and hence potentially on growth proved in this study to be whether a state set its income eligibility level for nursing home care equal to the level of maximum reimbursement it would pay a nursing home or lower than the reimbursement level. The former, presumably, provided easier access to nursing home care. Among the sample States, six were operating under the former setup at the beginning of the study period while only three—all northern States—were operating under the latter system. In those three States—New Jersey, South Dakota, and Vermont—all individuals whose incomes fell below the States' reimbursement rate for nursing home care but above the income eligibility level for welfare benefits were ineligible for coverage of nursing home care under the OAA, AABD, or MAA program, regardless of need. The particular system in place in each of the sample States had been set up with the adoption of one of these programs in the early 1960s. One exception—Mississippi—had no nursing home care program prior to 1967, at which point it adopted the "liberal" approach typical of southern states under OAA.

A number of factors which will be discussed later make it very difficult to trace the impact of the income eligibility determination process on the relative access to nursing home care available in a State and ultimately, though indirectly, on the pattern of nursing home growth which occurred there. One of these, the potential departure of application at the local level from State level policy, has already been mentioned. Another serious problem lies in the fact that except in South Dakota, where a switch from the "northern" to the "southern" approach was made under the same program (OAA) within the study period, and in Mississippi, which first adopted an OAA program in 1967, each State's system was in place at the beginning of the study period. Consequently, lacking anything but sketchy data on earlier years, we are unable to determine conclusively how this varied from what was in place earlier or what impact any changes may have had on the States' growth patterns at that point.

In South Dakota and Mississippi, much faster growth followed the adoption of a more "generous" eligibility system, but other concurrent developments there prevent an easy conclusion that these are causally linked. In Vermont and New Jersey, the other two States with the northern setup, growth was slow. In four of the six States with the more liberal arrangement in place at the beginning of the study period, it appears that easier access to nursing home care could have contributed to the rapid expansion of nursing home care which was taking place at that time.

Other components of eligibility policy must be considered as well. Limits on level of assets (principally savings) were identified as a deterrent to growth in one sample State, although, overall, asset limitation policy seems to have paralleled income policy in most States and does not seem to have exerted a significant independent impact. The same picture emerged with regard to limits placed on the transfer of property in order to attain eligibility status. Most States had imposed limits of from two to five years under programs in place at that time. Two other dimensions of eligibility policy—the imposition of liens on property and relative responsibility for contributions toward the maintenance of an assistance recipient—seem to have been practiced largely in the northeastern States. In two of these States—Vermont and New Jersey—these policies may well have functioned as deterrents to nursing home use. In all of the other sample States, at least, such policies either had been dropped, or if still on the books, went unenforced by the mid-1960s.

At this point some significant differences between the eligibility systems typical in the North or Northeast and those in the South should be mentioned. Those northern states opting for the more "liberal" income determination policy usually accomplished this through a medically needy/spend down provision. Southern states, which, it appears, almost always opted for the more "liberal" income approach, made the income cut-off level in effect equal to the nursing home reimbursement level by allowing the cost of nursing home care up to the state's reimbursement level to be included in the program applicant's budget— thus making many with incomes above the case assistance level but below the cost of nursing home care, categorically needy. Degree of liberality of income eligibility in those states setting the cut-off equal to the maximum reimbursement level, then, depended ultimately upon the level set for reimbursement.

Most southern states, however, did not reimburse nursing homes for the full difference between the recipient's income and the nursing home's charge to the recipient. The state, rather, depended upon the recipient's relatives or some charitable source to make up some of the difference. This arrangement, called "family supplementation," was reputed to have significantly constrained access to nursing home care in some states, and, as a consequence of court actions, was completely phased out by the end of the study period.

We were unable to establish that this policy exerted a highly significant impact in any of the southern States included in the sample. On the whole, it may have functioned as a less significant barrier to nursing home care than did relative responsibility policies enforced in some northern states.

Medical assessment for the purpose of determining nursing home care eligibility before 1970 was left up to the local caseworker and the applicant's attending physician in all of the sample States. As a result, it does not seem to have shaped access to nursing home care on a statewide or nationwide basis in any significant or consistent way up to that point. Only since 1970 (at the earliest) have states taken action to establish formal screening procedures with specialized staff assigned to this function. In only three of the sample States (Florida, New Jersey, and South Dakota) can these more formalized medical screening procedures be cited as even potentially negative influences on nursing home use at any point before the end of the study period. The principal impact of these procedures since 1972 generally has been a downgrading of many nursing home residents from SNF to ICF level status. Up to that point it is quite apparent that in most states, "assessment" typically resulted in a determination which reflected the need level covered by the state's major source of nursing home reimbursement.[1]

We have mentioned several factors which complicate the assessment of the impact of eligibility policy on nursing home growth over the past decade. One of these is state reimbursement policy. As we have seen, income eligibility for nursing home care throughout much of the study period, especially in southern states, was tied directly to reimbursement level. Reimbursement policy and its impacts upon nursing home growth is the subject to which we next turn our attention.

Reimbursement

Judging from the experience of the sample States, it appears that in the majority of cases changes in eligibility policy were accompanied by very significant changes in reimbursement policy. This was the case in five out of six sample States for which data availability allows us to make that determination. As has been pointed out, major revamping of eligibility policy in most States was undertaken simultaneously with and under the impetus of a state's adoption of a new medical assistance program. These new programs—OAA, AABD, MAA—most often brought with them the vendor method of payment and a significant rise in reimbursement. (The "vendor payment" method, in contrast to the "cash payment" method, involves submission of a bill or voucher by the provider to the government for service provided to the public program recipient and payment by the government directly to the provider without any intermediary action of the recipient. Third-party intermediaries such as Blue Cross-Blue Shield are used under the vendor method in some states, however.) In fact, it was not uncommon for reimbursement rates to be raised as a deliberate policy in order to stimulate a greater supply of nursing home beds to meet the expanded demand expected whenever eligibility was liberalized. Of course, increased federal matching rates also acted as an impetus to the adoption of higher rates.

This was in keeping with congressional intent, as increased federal match under these medical assistance programs was designed, in part, at least, to stimulate the expansion of nursing home care.

Until 1935, when OAA was enacted, the purchase of long-term care—aside from that provided by local governments for their pauperized populations housed in county poor farms and mental institutions—was entirely up to the individual. Even for the recipient of public funds, his or her monthly payment could be used for any purpose he or she decided, including the purchase of boarding house or nursing home care. Then, in 1950, for the first time the federal government authorized federal matching funds under the adult welfare titles for vendored payments to providers of medical care.

In 1956, this provision was liberalized by allowing the states federal matching funds determined on the basis of an average of all payments rather than on the basis of a monthly dollar ceiling per individual as had been required up to that point. This change in federal policy made it possible for states to cover large medical expenses such as nursing home care in more individual cases.

In spite of authorization and encouragement of vendor payments offered by legislation in 1950 and 1956, a significant number of states continued to use supplemental cash payments to welfare recipients for their care in nursing homes. In 1960, Congress again increased the incentive for states to use vendor payments through passage of the Kerr-Mills bill. This legislation authorized a higher federal match to states using vendor payments than to states making cash payments for medical care.

Those states adopting Medicaid in 1966 through 1969, of course, were required to use the vendor method for all medical payments funded under that program. By January 1970, all of the remaining states were required to adopt Medicaid programs or lose all federal participation in their medical assistance programs. This marked the end of all medical assistance under all welfare titles preceding Medicaid, although intermediate level care continued to be funded under Title XI until 1972, when it was placed under Title XIX (Medicaid) as well. Title XI of the Social Security Act had allowed the states to include nursing home care under one or all of their categorical assistance programs. OAA was most often used.

In addition to the change from cash payment to the vendor method of reimbursing nursing homes for publicly subsidized nursing home care in some states, a number of other developments in reimbursement took place over the course of the study decade. In many states that had not previously adopted such changes came uniform rates across counties, state rather than county adminis-tered payments, and treatment of the medical assistance rate as payment in full rather than as partial payment allowing for family supplementation. (States having such family supplementation arrangements were forced to phase them out in the early 1970s.)

In addition, adoption of the vendor payment method and the advent of the

Medical Assistance for the Aged and Medicaid programs brought at least a small increase in the federal share of the federal-state medical assistance costs. Under Medicaid, states were guaranteed a federal share of 105 percent of whatever federal share they received under their pre-Medicaid program. The maximum federal share also was raised to 83 percent, from 80 percent under MAA. (For a detailed description of the formulas and federal-state shares used under the OAA, MAA, and Medicaid programs, see appendix B.)

In part as a consequence, a number of states switched from facility-independent rates (flat rates) to cost-related reimbursement, and some of these, from reasonable cost with maximums to uncapped payment levels. Some also switched back to flat rates at some later point. Finally, all States raised their reimbursement levels and/or allowable costs at various points over the course of the study period.

Out of all of these changes, three—the adoption of the vendor payment method, the switch from facility-independent rates to cost-related reimbursement formulas, and the raising of the reimbursement per diem rates—appear to hold the greatest potential for explaining nursing home growth. These were the three most frequently cited by respondents as accounting for the observed expansion in their States.

Vendor Payments

The adoption of vendor payments was felt by some to have stimulated nursing home bed supply because it provided nursing homes for the first time with a reliable and uniform source of payment. The vendor method was adopted in New Jersey, New York, and Wisconsin prior to 1960. In Alabama, state vendor payments were introduced in 1960; in Florida, 1961; in California and Vermont, 1962; West Virginia, 1966; and in Mississippi and South Dakota, 1967.

The absence of pre-1960 data, including the exact year in which vendor payment mechanisms were adopted, in the first three sample States prevents their inclusion in any evaluation of the independent impact of the adoption of vendor payments on nursing home growth. Moreover, of the remaining seven States which adopted vendor payment mechanisms after 1960, we have annual bed supply growth figures for years preceding the adoption of the vendor payment method in only three—California, Mississippi, and South Dakota.

In California and Mississippi, we might note that the peak bed growth year within the study period occurred two and three years, respectively, after the adoption of the vendor payment program. South Dakota experienced two virtually equal peak years, the year before and the year immediately following the adoption of vendor payments in 1967. In two of the remaining four States, Alabama and Florida, the peak growth year appears to have occurred three years after adoption of the vendor program, although, as indicated, bed supply figures for years preceding the adoption of the vendor program are unavailable in those States, so that we cannot be certain of the rate of growth in those early years (see table 5-1).

As indicated above, the adoption of the vendor method of reimbursing nursing homes coincided variously with a number of other potentially significant developments, including a significant hike in the per diem rates nursing homes received. In fact, in six of the seven sample States for which we have data, the adoption of a vendor program was accompanied by an increase in reimbursement. Perhaps this is the reason that in only one sample State was the substitution of vendor for cash payments singled out specifically as responsible for a significant expansion in that State's bed supply.

In a number of States, adoption of the vendor method coincided with the very first viable nursing home program in those States. That is, it was established concurrently with the adoption of the OAA, AABD, or MAA program. Consequently, some of the impact associated with the adoption of a vendor payment mechanism could, in reality, reflect the effects of expanded eligibility, the setting up of screening procedures, and all that may have accompanied the fielding of these new programs. In the only State (South Dakota) in our sample which switched from cash payments to the vendor mechanism several years after entry into one of the formal nursing home programs, rapid growth preceded as well as followed the initiation of the vendor program.

Table 5-1
Status of Reimbursement Data and Key Policy Dates in the Ten Sample States

State	Year of Earliest Reimbursement Data	Year of Earliest Supply Data	Year of V.P. Adoption	Year of First Big Rate Increase	Year of Peak Growth Rate
Alabama	1960	1961	1960	1962	1963, 1964
California	1963	1960	1962	1962	1964
Florida	1961	1962	1961	1961	1964
Mississippi	1964	1963	1967	1967	1970
New Jersey	1964	1964	Pre-1960	1970 ?	1973[b] 13.2 1965[b] 10.2
New York	1966	1964	Pre-1960	?	1969[b]
South Dakota	1970	1960	1967	1967	1966 (21.9) 1968 (21.7)
Vermont	1963	1962	1962	Pre-1967 ? 1967	1973[a]
West Virginia	1960	1961	1966	1967	1974[a]
Wisconsin	1970	1964	Pre-1960	1967 ?	1965[b]

[a]Date missing or some bed data problem.

[b]Not considered in assessment of reimbursement rates and vendor payments because it could not be determined when the vendor payment method was adopted.

Reimbursement Methods

The use of a facility-independent rate rather than a facility cost-related formula for determining level of reimbursement has by and large characterized vendor payments to nursing homes. Such facility-independent rates have normally taken one of three forms: (1) a single statewide rate, (2) several statewide rates determined on the basis of care level or compliance with licensure standards (particularly fire safety), or (3) rates negotiated facility-by-facility or industry-wide at the county level. There were some exceptions to reliance on this mode of determining reimbursements, however. Some of the States which utilized MAA adopted policies of reimbursing facilities on the basis of their reasonable costs up to a maximum after that program was launched in 1960. Most States, by the end of the study period, continued to use either flat (facility-independent) rates or cost reimbursement with ceilings. Respondents in a number of instances informed us that the latter functioned similarly to flat rates in the sense that most facilities ended up receiving the same rate because their reported costs matched or exceeded the maximum rate the State would pay.

Nonetheless, respondents in eight out of ten States indicated that providers viewed cost-related reimbursement as more attractive than facility-independent rates, at least when it was first introduced in the States. It does appear to reduce the risk of investment; and where no maximum is imposed, it appears to guarantee that at least a provider's costs will be reimbursed. Cost reimbursement also would seem to offer opportunity for increased profits through loopholes in the rules by which providers are permitted to determine costs.

The method by which the reimbursement rate is determined—that is, reasonable cost, facility-independent rate, and so on—however, seems to have exerted very little impact on the decisions of providers or would-be providers with regard to expansion activity much before the latter 1960s. A number of respondents informed us that the typical operator of that period was less of a profit-maximizer than the type that has dominated nursing home operations since the adoption of Medicaid and Medicare in the late 1960s. As a result, rates that were adequate though not necessarily highly profitable may have been sufficient to stimulate a rather significant expansion in the bed supply. The absence of vigorous standards enforcement prior to 1970 undoubtedly also made it easier to do reasonably well financially under the facility-independent rates which dominated at that time.

Provider response since the mid-1960s has been more complex than under predecessor programs. Nursing home operators became more financially sophisticated, responding, we were told, to seemingly minor changes in reimbursement *methods* as well as rates, and anticipating policy changes (and, through lobbying efforts, helping to bring about such changes) rather than simply reacting to them after the fact.

Yet no consistent pattern in terms of the impact of reimbursement methods since the mid-1960s emerged in our analysis, even within States grouped by type of policy. For example, three States in the sample—Alabama, Vermont, and Wisconsin—reimbursed nursing homes on an uncapped, cost-related basis. In Alabama adoption of this policy was followed by bed supply growth. In Vermont the implementation of uncapped cost reimbursement was followed (temporarily) by depressed growth and can be said to be related to supply growth only if one accepts as reasonable a four-year lag between policy change and supply response. A change to the reasonable cost reimbursement method in Wisconsin was unmarked by any discernible shift in supply pattern.

Similarly, among the six sample States which adopted a reasonable cost with a ceiling reimbursement system under Medicaid in the late 1960s, no pattern emerges clearly. In New Jersey, New York, and South Dakota, this switch in reimbursement method was followed by more rapid bed supply expansion, but an apparent decline in the attractiveness of the reimbursement rate (due to small increases in the maximums, or changes in the formula) thereafter was blamed for a slowdown in expansion. And in California, cost-related reimbursements were viewed by the nursing home industry as less attractive than the modified flat rates they replaced, with the reported result that such reimbursement policy served to constrain growth. Similarly, no clear patterns emerged from groupings of the sample States by region, Medicaid adoption date, size, or "sophistication." Perhaps the cost-related method of establishing the reimbursement rate does not have the clear-cut advantages to the provider that it is often assumed to have.

It seems likely that the great variation in cost-related approaches makes any generalization about the relative advantage of such a method versus flat-rate determination risky. Those formulas which impose no ceiling on costs or which provide significant loopholes for cost determination may very well be preferred over flat rates, while those with low ceilings or those which are monitored closely will appear less attractive to providers. The reported enthusiasm for the cost-related method among providers may reflect in no small part the fact that payments determined under a cost-based formula have usually been higher than those that had existed under the facility-independent method which preceded it. It may very well be that, for any given reimbursement level, providers in general would prefer the facility-independent approach because it involves no cost reporting or justification requirements often imposed under cost-related systems.

Reimbursement Rates

As indicated in the discussion of reimbursement policy, the supply of nursing homes in each State before the latter 1960s appears to have been fairly responsive to the level of payment regardless of the system of rate determination in use. Most States, however, did in fact employ facility-independent rates or, in a few instances, rates based on a point system at that time.

Although, for understandable reasons, respondents were often unable to separate the impacts of these separate components of reimbursement policy, reimbursement levels or rate increases were cited most frequently as aspects of reimbursement exerting the most direct impact on bed expansion. In fact, of all the policy variables discussed, an increase in reimbursement level was mentioned most frequently as the key reason for growth in nursing home bed supply. Overall, however, it appears to have exerted more direct or visible impact earlier in the study period than later. By the early 1970s and certainly by the close of the study period, the impact of reimbursement seems to have become somewhat muted by the interactive effects of other policies, especially licensure enforcement and, increasingly, planning and direct controls over the entry of providers.

For the reasons discussed—namely, simultaneity of several policy changes and lack of key data as well as developments in eligibility policy—it is impossible with the study approach employed here to determine in any conclusive way the single aspect of nursing home reimbursement which exerted the greatest influence on provider decisions. On the basis of respondent perception, however, as well as our own "gestalt" reading of events in ten States, it appears that level of reimbursement is the key facet of reimbursement policy to consider in any explanation of growth in the nursing home bed supply in recent decades. This "judgment call" is assisted somewhat by the observation of Thomas that the vendor payment mechanism in itself was of minor importance, at least in New York State.[2]

Capital Funding

Among the variables considered in this study for their potential impact on nursing home growth in the United States over the past decade, the availability of capital funding probably is the most difficult to assess because of the dearth of relevant information available from State or federal sources. Specifically, we were interested in the effects on nursing home growth over the study period of the availability of commercial loans, Federal Housing Authority (FHA) loan guarantees, Small Business Administration (SBA) loans, Hill-Burton grants and loans, and special state funding mechanisms. From what we were able to learn from State respondents and federal officials (as well as from the fact that all of the federal subsidy programs are locally administered) it appears that the volume of use of the federal funding subsidies as well as the ease with which commercial loans could be obtained varied significantly by state and over time.

Commercial Loans

The most frequently used funding source, it appears, was the commercial loan. As might be expected, however, data on these are the most difficult to come by.

In only two States—Florida and South Dakota—was difficulty in obtaining bank loans cited by respondents as particularly important in affecting nursing home bed expansion during any part of the study period. It is quite clear from responses of State officials, including nursing home association spokesmen, however, that commercial loans were difficult to obtain in the early years of the study period before nursing homes were determined to be a reliable investment. Nursing homes suffered from being viewed by lenders as buildings of single-purpose construction and hence unusable for other purposes in the event the nursing home venture failed. The introduction of Medicaid and Medicare appears to have further solidified the position of nursing homes as reliable investments, although in a few places, such as California, the overbuilding and low occupancy rates which resulted from the shifts in Medicare policy in 1969 almost surely damaged the image of nursing homes as an investment and made loans once again very difficult to obtain, at least in those parts of the State where overbuilding had occurred. See chapter 7 for a description of those shifts in Medicare policy.

The relative availability of commercial loans also seems tied to reimbursements such that when reimbursement is unattractive (or policy unpredictable) and hence less likely to cover costs or produce a reasonable profit, banks and loan associations are less likely to approve a loan. Respondents in Florida noted that this was the situation in that State when reimbursements slipped and policy fluctuated wildly in the latter part of the study period.

It should be noted that the early 1970s were marked by high interest rates throughout the national economy, so that loans for money to construct or expand nursing home operations, like other businesses, were difficult to obtain. This factor no doubt contributed in some measure to lowering the overall growth rate of the nursing home industry during the last segment of the study decade.

FHA

Federal Housing Administration (FHA) mortgage guarantees became available through the Housing Act of 1959 for the construction of for-profit skilled nursing homes. Amendments to the 1964 and 1969 Housing Acts extended availability to private, nonprofit skilled and intermediate care facilities. They have been of particular help to the proprietary nursing home sector and, with the possible exception of Hill-Burton monies, comprise the most important source of federal assistance for nursing home expansion. On the basis of respondent reports, it would appear that the availability or use of FHA loan guarantees has been of some, though not necessarily great, importance in shaping growth patterns at some point in four of the sample States—Mississippi, New York, South Dakota, and Wisconsin. A somewhat different picture emerges from table 5-2, which shows in the second column the number of FHA-insured beds per

Table 5-2
Volume of FHA-Insured Mortgages for Nursing Homes under Title II, Section 232, in Sample States, 1935-1974

	Number of Beds	Number of FHA Beds/ 100 Elderly (1970)	Number of FHA Insurance Beds/ Number of Beds (1974)
U.S.	110,485	0.55	0.10 (1973)
Alabama	819	0.25	0.05
California	7,197	NA[a]	0.07
Florida	4,897	NA[a]	0.16
Mississippi	1,784	0.81	0.20
New Jersey	8,091	1.17	0.32
New York	13,048	0.67	0.15
South Dakota	167	0.21	0.02
Vermont	914	1.94	0.30
West Virginia	756	0.39	0.24
Wisconsin	3,403	0.72	0.07

Source: U.S. Department of Housing and Urban Development, *1974 Statistical Yearbook* (Washington, D.C.: United States Government Printing Office, 1974) Table 141, p. 136.
[a]NA = Not Available.

100 elderly population in the sample States. Mississippi and Wisconsin show up as high users, while New Jersey and Vermont emerge as higher users than New York or South Dakota. Respondents in both New Jersey and Vermont indicated that FHA had guaranteed "at least a few mortgages" in the early years of the study period. It is, of course, often difficult for respondents to reconstruct the past accurately, particularly when a number of forces seem to have been (and likely were) shaping the nursing home scene simultaneously.

There is little question that the importance of FHA mortgage guarantees varied over both time and locale. The necessity of obtaining a loan guarantee in order to acquire a commercial loan seems to have been present in most places during the earlier portion of the study period when nursing homes were viewed rather widely as risky investments. At the same time, however, large loans were less often needed because many nursing homes were converted family dwellings.

Variability across localities in access to FHA loan guarantees perhaps could be assumed from the fact that the program is administered through local offices scattered throughout the country. Although no hard data are available with which to confirm this, a knowledgeable official in the FHA central office, as well as State officials, believe that these local offices varied significantly in their application requirements and in their willingness to approve guarantees for nursing home loans during the period covered in this study.

SBA

Small Business Administration (SBA) loans first became available to nursing home builders in 1956, but they have never been used to any significant degree.

Apparently they have never been considered attractive to nursing home investors because of the relatively low loan ceiling of $350,000, and the short mortgage period of only ten years allowed by the program.[3] Respondents in only one sample State, South Dakota, indicated that SBA had supplied "quite a few" loans.

State Programs

Special state programs for funding nursing home construction were established during the study period in only two of the sample States, Alabama and New York. Under both programs, municipalities were encouraged to float tax-free bonds, the income from which could be loaned at low interest rates to nonprofit enterprises seeking to construct a medical facility. In Alabama, the main objective of the program was to expand acute care facilities. Because of this and because it was available only to nonprofit providers, its impact on Alabama's rapid growth appears to have been modest at best, even though the program existed from the beginning of the study period. New York's program, set up in 1967, on the other hand, was expressly designed to encourage nursing home expansion in the nonprofit sector and seems to have played a highly significant role in the growth spurt New York experienced in the early 1970s.

Information available from our forty-four-state phone survey indicates that only a few states had special funding programs in place during any part of the study decade. Consequently, they seem largely unrelated to the overall nursing home growth which this country experienced over that period.

Hill-Burton

The second major, though relatively small, source of capital subsidization was the Hill-Burton program. Enacted in 1946 as the Hospital Survey and Construction Act, it was designed to foster the expansion of public hospitals, through the offering of construction grants, particularly in rural areas lacking medical facilities. An amendment to the program in 1954, the Medical Facilities Survey and Construction Act, made construction grants available for the first time to nonprofit nursing homes. These federal funds were allocated to states on the basis of population size and wealth (through a formula that favored rural states) and were distributed to individual projects through state Hill-Burton agencies housed in state health departments. In 1969 the grant program was replaced with a much less popular loan subsidy program called Hill-Harris. The program as such was phased out entirely in 1974 with passage of the Health Planning and Resources Development Act.[4] Cumulative grants to nursing homes from July 1947 to June 1971 totaled $171,648,000. In all, 37,884 nursing home beds were constructed with Hill-Burton monies over that period.[5]

The direct impact of the Hill-Burton program on nursing home bed supply has been modest. In part, this is due to the fact that it could be used only for nonprofit operations in an industry that is very dominantly proprietary. Then, too, appropriations under the Community Health Services and Facilities Act did not keep pace with congressional authorizations so that funding levels imposed a limitation on its use. Some of the funds could be and were used for purposes other than addition of beds—for example, modification or additions to dining halls or laundry facilities. Some states funneled their funds almost exclusively into expansion of acute care, while a significant number of hospitals used Hill-Burton long-term care grants to construct long-term care beds and then, at the first opportunity, converted these beds to acute care use. Time consumed in processing grant applications as well as the Davis-Bacon and indigent support requirements also may have played a role in reducing program utilization.

In keeping with the design of the original program, Hill-Burton monies have exerted the greatest impact on nursing home bed capacity in rural states, especially those in the north central region of the country. Among the sample States, Hill-Burton funding appears to have been especially important in explaining growth in South Dakota. It appears to have gained high usage there because of the tradition of sectarian and community sponsorship and operation of medical facilities, and because the state Hill-Burton agency actively encouraged the use of such funding by communities for the construction of nursing homes rather than hospital beds.

The real importance of the Hill-Burton program lies not in its direct impact on bed supply but rather in the influence it has exerted on nursing home licensure standards, on the notion of bed need (and hence on the feasibility decisions of moneylenders with respect to nursing home loan applications), and on health planning. These dimensions of nursing home policy, in turn, have come to impact rather directly on bed supply. Regulation of the nursing home industry through licensure and certification standards, planning, and direct controls on capital expansion is the subject of the next chapter.

Notes

1. See, for example, William Thomas, Jr., *Nursing Homes and Public Policy* (Ithaca: Cornell University Press, 1969), p. 87.

2. Thomas, p. 96.

3. Thomas, p. 174.

4. For a very informative discussion of the Hill-Burton program, see Thomas, especially pp. 111-120.

5. Judith R. Fave and Lester B. Fave, *The Hospital Construction Act* (Washington, D.C.: American Enterprise Institute for Public Policy Research, 1974), p. 14.

6

Regulation of the Nursing Home Industry

Not surprisingly, the sequel to governmental subsidization of nursing home care has been governmental regulation. In this chapter we review the principal efforts taken by governmental policymakers to insure that the government (and presumably the American citizenry) was getting its money's worth out of the expenditures it was making to provide nursing home care to public patients. The key efforts have centered in licensure and certification of facilities, and in planning and regulation of bed stock expansion. For a detailed description of standards applicable under each of the federal subsidy programs, including a timeline of such standards, see appendix B.

Licensure and Certification Standards and Their Enforcement

Licensure of nursing homes has always been a state health department function. Federal certification has been required of facilities receiving federal funds only since the implementation of the Medicare and Medicaid programs. The certifying process is carried out by states (usually health departments) under contract with the U.S. Department of Health, Education and Welfare. Usually, the inspections or surveys of facilities for certification and licensure purposes are conducted by the same inspectors simultaneously. The two processes are treated together here for the latter part of the study period since the vast majority of licensed nursing homes are also certified for Medicaid and/or Medicare participation. In fact, as of 1974, only 23 percent of facilities and only 14 percent of the beds in this country's nursing homes remained uncertified.[1] In some of the less wealthy states—for example, Vermont, Alabama, and Mississippi—the proportion of licensed facilities that are also certified approaches 100 percent.

However, the development of state licensing standards as well as their enforcement has come largely as a consequence of federal initiative. The earliest standards in most states appeared around 1950 with the adoption of the Old Age Assistance program. After 1953, under this program, a state could receive matching federal funds only if it agreed to establish a standard-setting mechanism under the auspices of the state health department and to develop some nursing home standards, the content of which was left to the states. A number of states latched onto the Hill-Burton conforming standards for newly constructed facilities as a model when that funding program first became available for the construction of nursing homes in 1954. By and large, however, standards adopted by the states were minimal and focused almost exclusively on the physical plant—that is, sanitation and safety.

In no state, apparently, were Hill-Burton physical standards applied this early to existing facilities, but only to facilities constructed after these standards were adopted. From both our sample State case studies and our telephone survey, it became clear that the Life Safety Code and other physical standards were not enforced in older facilities until the early 1970s. In fact, in many states, it appears that periodic, systematic inspections of nursing homes were the exception rather than the rule before 1970, when final federal certification standards for skilled nursing homes participating in the Medicaid program became enforceable for the first time.

The period 1964 through 1966 in large measure marked the transition to the modern nursing home. This was the time during which many states adopted new sets of standards which were significantly more rigorous, especially with regard to fire safety, than those that existed prior to that point. The impetus for this activity undoubtedly varied from state to state. In a few States, such as California and Florida, the passage of new legislation authorizing the tougher standards seems to have grown to some degree out of a desire of the licensing bureaus in the State health departments to improve the quality of nursing home care, or at least to lessen the risk of nursing home fires. In some States, such as California and Vermont, facilities which met the physical standards for licensure received a higher reimbursement level under the Old Age Assistance or Medical Assistance for the Aged program than did nonconforming facilities. There is no evidence, however, that facilities which failed to meet state standards anywhere were closed for that reason. The experience of the sample States strongly suggests that reimbursement levels were too low, demand for beds was too great, and the enforcement resources of state licensing agencies were too meager to make anything resembling vigorous enforcement a reality.

The first federal standards imposed on nursing homes (aside from Hill-Burton funded facilities) came as a result of the passage of the Medicare Extended Care Facility program in 1965. This program became operational in the states in 1967. With the establishment of this program, federal standards affecting patient care were prescribed for those facilities which were able to participate in the program. Staffing standards were promulgated for ECFs in May 1966. The Life Safety Code was not included in the regulations until 1971. The pressure from HEW to make this program a success—that is, to obtain a large supply of beds in nursing homes designated as Extended Care Facilities— however, resulted in many states in the certification of (making eligible for program participation) any facility that was state licensed, regardless of the fact that most states at that time had very weak licensure enforcement programs.

Except for Hill-Burton facilities and Medicare-certified ECFs, serious en- forcement of standards affecting patient care (staffing standards, handling of drugs, patient records, and the like) has evolved only since 1970. The same is true of physical construction standards applied to existing facilities, which were grandfathered into federal program participation by virtue of state licensure status. Significantly more demanding federal regulations in homes certified as "skilled nursing homes" (SNHs) and later as "skilled nursing facilities" (SNFs) than had been applied to most nursing homes (except Hill-Burton and Medicare certified homes) became enforceable under the Medicaid program at that point.

In general, enforcement of standards for nursing homes of the type commonly first certified for Medicaid participation as "intermediate care facilities" (ICFs) did not begin until 1974, when different federal standards for ICFs became enforceable and 100 percent federal funding for all certification costs was made available to the states. At that point many states doubled or tripled the size of their inspection staffs, making, for the first time, systematic annual inspections of nursing home facilities feasible. This became possible because much of the inspection process could be completed simultaneously by the same staff for both federal certification and state licensure purposes.

The direct impact of licensure and certification activities on nursing home growth over the relatively brief study period are difficult to summarize. Part of the problem stems from the fact that changes in state licensure and certification activities were almost always accompanied by simultaneous changes in other state policies affecting nursing homes—most notably, reimbursement policies and often planning policies as well. Moreover, the direction of impact in terms of growth in bed stock of standards enforcement seems to have varied other both time and place. Then, too, standards have to do with both those structures or procedures directly affecting patient care and those requirements applied to the physical setting in which the care is rendered. Of these, standards affecting the physical setting appear to have had the most discernible effect.

Obviously, a step-up in enforcement of standards can retard growth through the decertification or closure of substandard facilities, thereby removing units from the bed stock. In facilities dependent upon Medicaid patients, decertification can be tantamount to removal of an operating license. This happened, as indicated, largely after 1970, with the emergence of final federal regulation applicable to skilled nursing homes; although many facilities which failed to meet skilled standards at that time were downgraded to a lower certification or licensure category—often to ICF status—at least until final federal standards applicable to ICFs were promulgated in 1974. Even then, retention in the program rather than decertification (which in a significant number of cases leads to closure) seems to have been assisted in some places by the authority of states, delegated by HEW regional offices, to grant waivers to skilled facilities falling short in some of the standards. Waiver-granting authority for ICFs was retained by the states when Medicaid coverage was made available to cover ICF care in 1972, so that the impact on closures of the 1974 federal ICF standards seems to have been somewhat mitigated in many states.

Facility closure or decertification is typically a long and drawn-out process fraught with legal battles and maneuvers, often putting the state licensure agency or state's attorney handling such cases at a distinct disadvantage because of the lack of legal resources commonly available to state regulatory agencies. Nevertheless, the slowdown in nursing home growth which has occurred since the end of the study period may reflect, in some part, the effects of the imposition of the 1974 standards in ICFs. Up to that point, it was possible to prevent the loss of much needed nursing home beds when facilities could no longer pass the standards for SNF certification—especially the Life Safety Code imposed in 1970—by converting them to ICF status. However, since 1974, many of these small, converted family dwellings will have had to upgrade their facilities, close, or downgrade to personal care home status—then ceasing to be included in state's nursing home bed stock. Thus, the most significant single effect of standards enforcement on the supply of nursing home beds may well have occurred just after the study decade ended and thus will begin to show up in nursing home bed statistics in the 1976 NCHS survey. At the same time, it appears that a substantial number of "substandard" ICFs continue to be licensed and certified in many, if not most, states.

No impact of licensure and certification activities on nursing home growth patterns during the study period was discernible in three of the ten sample States—Alabama, Florida, and West Virginia. Of the remaining States, five— California, New Jersey, Mississippi, Vermont. and Wisconsin—all experienced temporary and rather sudden drops in their rates of growth of nursing home bed supply as a result, at least in part, of facility closures. This came in the early 1970s with federally mandated enforcement of the Life Safety Code in SNFs. These drops in growth were followed in some States—for example, Vermont, where the pattern was especially clear-cut—by particularly rapid expansion in bed stocks owing to the replacement of these typically small homes with much larger facilities.

Standards enforcement also can retard growth by making the construction and operation of nursing homes more expensive, leading to a reduction in the number of provider applicants and/or an increase in the number of operators who close down their facilities. Both results have occurred, although the former has probably had more impact. A health department official in Wisconsin informed us that a very noticeable decline in the number of applications for a license to operate a nursing home occurred after the enactment in 1964 of a new set of much more rigorous standards, containing staffing as well as automatic-sprinklering requirements.

In sum, at the same time that standards enforcement activities have functioned to lessen the size of the nursing home bed stock through forced and voluntary facility closures and through increased construction costs which discourage potential providers, they also have indirectly led to growth through the replacement of older, smaller facilities with new ones, containing many more beds. Although no satisfactory way exists to measure it quantitatively, the net effect of standards enforcement functioning through this replacement mechanism may well constitute at least a slight plus over the study period.

Although impossible to measure tangibly with existing data, there is little doubt that standards enforcement has contributed to the expansion of nursing home care also because, on the whole, it has made nursing homes much more attractive and acceptable settings to place impaired persons in. Not only are today's nursing homes very often more physically attractive than many of the old, two-story, wooden-frame structures which they replaced, but the Life Safety Code has made them from all appearances into safe residences. Maybe even more important, enforcement of standards affecting patient care has made nursing homes more and more acceptable components of the medical care system. The presence of nurses, pharmacies, medical charts, and nurses' stations has transformed nursing homes into medical settings. As a result, physicians as well as consumers are more inclined to use then for patients requiring recuperative care following acute episodes as well as for persons needing chronic care. In sum, more vigorous standards enforcement over the course of the study period, beginning in a few places as early as 1964, but especially since 1970, appears to have improved the perception of nursing homes among the general population and among physicians, increasing their legitimacy.

One thing is certain. Increased regulation of the nursing home industry over the course of the past decade has contributed immensely to the transformation of that industry. The typical nursing home as we know it at the end of the study period was an exception in 1964. In 1964, the typical nursing home was an older, wooden-frame, two- or three-story converted house, containing perhaps forty beds, owned and operated by a husband and wife, with an LPN supervising staff activities during the day shift. Today, the Life Safety Code with its expensive provisions and the information and reporting requirements for participation in federal funding programs—principally Medicaid—has produced typically a single-story, fire-resistive facility of sixty beds frequently owned by a corporation or partnership of investors and often managed by a salaried nursing home administrator. It houses a larger proportion of sicker patients and employs RNs and/or LPNs supervising staff functions on all shifts. Costs imposed by these standards have made a large operation economically necessary. This form of operation, in turn, has converted nursing homes into settings that, though physically attractive, resemble more the higher-regimented, impersonal, acute care hospital than the more familylike residential settings of a decade or two ago. Of course, in states that had made heavy use of Hill-Burton monies for the construction of nursing homes and that had imposed Hill-Burton physical standards on newly constructed facilities by the later 1950s, there were already in 1964 a significant number of "modern" facilities.

Whether this transformation would have occurred without federal initiative is a moot question, perhaps. It is clear that action in most states was taken in direct response to the initiation of a new federal funding program for long-term care through which states could multiply state dollars—first OAA and Hill-Burton, then MAA and finally Medicare and Medicaid. In a few states, concern for improved quality of care seems to have arisen somewhat independently. Be that as it may, we can be quite certain that the transformation which has occurred would not have come as early without federal initiative.

Although standards enforcement contributed greatly to shaping of the nursing home industry over the course of the study decade, the impact of this factor on both growth of nursing home care and the transformation of that care mode as previously indicated did not, for the most part, occur independently of the impacts of other developments—most notably, reimbursement policy. One conclusion regarding standards enforcement that emerges from this study is that the rigor of enforcement has been closely correlated with the willingness of the state to pay for the facilities' cost of meeting these standards through the reimbursement mechanism for public pay patients. Recognizing the close connection between compliance with standards and the level of reimbursement, states sometimes raised reimbursement levels whenever new standards required expensive improvements. Moreover, it appears that most states undertook to *enforce* standards only when they were in a position to pay nursing homes enough for the facility to be able to absorb the costs of complying with the standards.

Special Impact of the Hill-Burton Program on Nursing Home Standards

Eligibility for Hill-Burton funding carried the requirement that a facility meet a series of unprecedented, high-level standards. These standards pertained to both the physical structure of the facility and to the patient care delivered therein. The physical standards required that a facility be structurally sound and fire safe. They were quite specific and resembled the Life Safety Code standards as we know them today. In addition, all certified Hill-Burton facilities were required to have twenty-four-hour supervision of patients by a registered nurse. To ensure enforcement of these standards, states, of course, were required to have a nursing home licensure apparatus in place.

These new standards imposed under Hill-Burton were a far cry from anything that had existed for nursing homes up to that point. Beginning in the early 1950s, most states passed licensure laws and designated a nursing home licensing agency in order to receive federal OAA funds; but in almost all instances, these licensure laws were very general and vague, pertained largely to sanitation and physical structure, and were at best feebly enforced. As a consequence, the new Hill-Burton standards provided the earliest model of what, it was assumed in the vacuum that prevailed at that time, nursing home standards should be. This was reinforced by the distinction between number of conforming and number of nonconforming beds required in the annual Hill-Burton plan.

Thus, a number of states in the late 1950s and early 1960s enacted new licensure codes that closely resembled the Hill-Burton standards, especially with regard to fire safety provisions. For example, New York in 1961 passed a law requiring that *all* nursing home construction projects be in substantial compliance with Hill-Burton standards before being approved. This, of course, greatly increased the cost of construction and undoubtedly reduced the number of provider applicants. A few states also followed the lead of Hill-Burton standards by including at least some minimal staffing requirements in their new licensure codes commonly enacted in the early or mid-1960s. Rarely were such standards as specific as the twenty-four-hour supervisory RN required under Hill-Burton. Nonetheless, this Hill-Burton standard reinforced among state health officials the idea that specific standards should be applied to nursing homes.

By viewing nursing homes as medical facilities and thereby imposing on nursing homes conditions of participation in the Hill-Burton program that were decidedly hospital and physician-oriented—and that served in many respects as models for both federal and state regulations later on—the Public Health Service firmly established the "medical model" as the appropriate one for nursing homes. In fact, Hill-Burton funding decisions have favored hospital-based facilities and have required that all nonhospital-based facilities affiliate themselves with a general hospital through a written agreement for transfer of patients and use of staff. (See Thomas for a discussion of this Public Health Service orientation.)[2] The "medical model" continues today to dominate public policy toward long-term care of the elderly.

According to Thomas, the biggest contribution of the Hill-Burton program was the administrative idea it introduced of a broad organizational (systems) perspective specified by the rational organization of health care institutions—for example, nursing homes in relation to hospitals—on a communitywide basis.[3] This was the planning idea and the beginning of comprehensive health planning and regulation of provider entry—subjects to which we turn our attention in the next section of this study.

Health Facility Planning and Regulation of Capital Expansion

To ensure that Hill-Burton funded projects were built where they were most needed, state Hill-Burton agencies were required to produce an annual facilities construction plan which contained estimates of skilled nursing bed needs for each planning region of the state. These estimates were made on the basis of a bed-need estimating formula adopted by the Public Health Service. Several variations of this formula have been used, but basically the formula made use of the past year's utilization rate (beds per 1,000 persons sixty-five years of age and older) and projected growth in the size of the elderly population to estimate bed need three to five years ahead. Theoretically, at least, these estimates were then compared with existing and conforming bed stocks in those regions by the Hill-Burton agencies and used to allocate Hill-Burton funds among the planning regions of the state.

The state plans which contained the nursing home bed-need estimates were viewed primarily by state health officials as fund-allocating devices rather than planning documents. Nonetheless, they functioned to introduce an initial technique for regulating the supply of long-term care beds.

The early influence of Hill-Burton estimates (soon after the program was implemented) at the state level on the supply of nursing home beds came about not through any formal design of state health departments but through the use of these estimates by capital funding sources to decide the feasibility of nursing home construction for which a mortage loan or guarantee was sought. Both FHA and SBA programs required that each applicant obtain from the state health department a certificate indicating that the proposed beds were needed in the area in which they were planned.[4] Private lenders, likewise, often used these estimates as guides in their feasibility studies of loan requests.

Rarely in the mid-1960s, however, does this process appear to have functioned to constrain supply. In very few areas was the bed stock anywhere near the level perceived as needed. Wherever the elderly population was growing, or wherever utilization rates were increasing, application of the Hill-Burton formula projected increased need. The Hill-Burton program, moreover, was directed at replacing substandard facilities with facilities that conformed to Hill-Burton construction standards. Thus, replacement was always needed for a substantial number of facilities. Besides, states were not required to follow the Hill-Burton formula religiously so that they were left with relatively broad discretion in determining need.

Many agencies—if not most—took other factors into account, and by the late 1960s some states were using this informal certificate-of-need process that developed to replace older non-fire-resistive facilities with new homes that met the stiffer state licensing standards. They simply let it be known through the publication of the Hill-Burton plan that a large number of new conforming beds would be needed.

Providing reimbursement rates were attractive, this usually resulted in a net increase in the bed supply because the replacement facilities were almost always larger. Moreover, in some places such as Vermont, the facilities which were to be replaced were determined later (after the replacement facilities had been built and added to the bed stock) to be in conformity with state standards and allowed to remain as well. Thus in that State, a substantial part of the surge in bed stock growth occurring in the early 1970s was in part traceable to state bed-need estimating policy.

Desire of the state health department to replace older homes with new fire-resistant facilities often resulted in giving the proprietary sector an advantage over the nonprofit sector, it seems. Because departments wanted to replace facilities as quickly as possible, they were quick to approve applications for construction. Because of their typically more cumbersome administrative and fund-raising mechanisms, several State licensure officials informed us, nonprofit providers, on average, take considerably longer to move on the application and construction process than do proprietary interests. As a consequence, it appears, the latter—once need estimates were published—moved in quickly with their formal plans to meet almost all of the anticipated bed shortage in a particular area before the nonprofits were ready to submit an application.

Partnership for Health Act

The Hill-Burton method of estimating bed need was carried over by and large into the federal government's first attempt to plan and regulate the nation's health services, including long-term care. This came with passage of the Partnership for Health Act of 1966 (P.L. 89-749). Under this law, local and state planning agencies were set up not only to plan services, but to participate in the facilities construction review function which the Hill-Burton agencies had come to perform. Lacking real teeth, these comprehensive planning agencies were forced to rely by and large upon voluntary compliance with their need determinations and thus were rarely effective in controlling provider behavior.

Section 1122

These state and local Comprehensive Health Planning Agencies took on added importance with passage of the 1972 Social Security Amendments, which for the first time authorized financial sanctions against facilities failing to comply with the decisions of the comprehensive planning agencies. Section 1122 of the 1972 amendment provided that any facility which made a capital expenditure of more than $100,000 or changed its services substantially without first obtaining the approval of the planning agencies would not be reimbursed under Titles V, XVIII, or XIX for that portion of their costs represented by the interest and depreciation of those unauthorized capital expenditures or by the provision of the unapproved services. This, of course, provided only partial certificate of need coverage of nursing home services, since only Medicare and Medicaid certified facilities and only reimbursement rather than licensing or certification status were affected. Moreover, adoption of an 1122 program was not made mandatory. Nonetheless, Medicaid is a most important source of funding for nursing homes. In some poorer states, all licensed homes participate in Medicaid.

The federal carrot offered to states to entice them to set up an 1122 review was increased planning funds. As of April 1, 1974, thirty-seven states had contracted with HEW to carry out 1122 reviews. Seven of the ten sample States had 1122 programs by the end of the study period. Since the program was not implemented anywhere except in Alabama until 1973, however, it obviously exerted little influence on the overall growth pattern observed for that decade. The initiation of an 1122 review process in Alabama in 1972 does appear to have contributed to a moderate growth spurt in 1973 as existing providers rushed in to grab up all the certificates as soon as the program went into effect in order to keep out competition.

Certificate of Need

In the 1974 Health Planning and Resource Development Act (P.L. 93-641), the federal government carried health care provider regulation a step further in requiring that all states establish a certificate-of-need program. Progress in getting all states to comply with this congressional mandate has been slow, however. Unlike the 1122 program, which in most states could be implemented administratively, a full-fledged certificate-of-need program which determines whether or not a would-be provider receives an operating license to open his facility, or facility addition, requires state enabling legislation. As of mid-1977, eighteen states had no certificate-of-need program in place.

Twenty-four states had passed the necessary state statutes and had programs operating as of April 1, 1974.[5] New York, one of our sample States, was the first to establish a program in 1966. Two other sample States, California and New Jersey, established programs in 1970 and 1971, respectively. California's program actually was not a full-fledged certificate-of-need program as we have defined it here, because it was used only to determine Medicaid and Medicare certification status. However, it was much more stringent than 1122 since it determined whether or not a facility could admit any Medicare or Medicaid patients, rather than just affecting a relatively small portion of a facility's reimbursement.

As was the case with the establishment of the 1122 program in Alabama, the enactment of certificate-of-need programs in California and New York appears to have produced an initial spurt in growth as providers there sped up their expansion activities in order to beat the deadline for the effective date of the program (as in California) or to grab up the initial certificates available in order to keep our future competition, and to hedge against an almost certain diminution in availability of franchises as existing bed needs were met.

Determination of the longer-range effect of certificates-of-need in these two

States is greatly encumbered by concurrent developments, principally changes in attractiveness of Medicaid reimbursement and, in California, low occupancy rates—and by different objectives for which the program was used. In California, which sought to put a lid on nursing home expansion, the program (after its initial stimulative effect) seems to have played an important role in constraining growth throughout the remainder of the study period. New York health officials, on the other hand, were most concerned with replacing substandard homes with conforming facilities so that they granted franchises for the construction of new beds rather liberally through 1973.

Respondents in New Jersey made no mention of any initial impact of certificate-of-need enactment in 1971, although that state experienced virtually no growth in 1972. The effect of the moratorium on issuance of certificates imposed from 1973 to mid-1975 was a negative growth rate from 1973 to 1974. Florida and South Dakota enacted certificate-of-need programs in 1973. Apparent loopholes in the Florida program rendered it inconsequential in impact on bed supply growth over the last year of the study period. Florida had been experiencing negative growth since 1969 anyway. Respondents in South Dakota claimed that their program has had a significantly negative impact on growth since its enactment. Negative growth experienced there between 1973 and 1974 supports this contention, although the absence of bed stock figures for years since 1974 prevents independent observation of impact since that point. It is interesting to note that South Dakota, like California, experienced a moderate growth surge in the same year that certificate-of-need was enacted.

Overall, given the recent time frame of most certificate-of-need programs, the fact that a significant proportion of states did not have programs during any part of the study period, and the very real possibility that some states used their programs to "stimulate" supply while others used them to slow expansion, it is clear that formal certificate-of-need programs do not help much in explaining the national pattern of nursing home growth over the study decade. They may help to explain the continued preponderance of skilled beds in New York and California, however. Apparently fearing that the certificate-of-need program will make it exceedingly difficult to ever acquire or regain SNF status for their beds once they are certified for a lower care level, nursing home operators are very reluctant to opt for less than skilled status.

Notes

1. Alvin Sirocco and Hugh Koch, "Nursing Homes in the United States, 1973-1974," *Vital and Health Statistics*, Series 14, No. 17, National Center for Health Statistics, U.S. Department of Health, Education and Welfare, 1977, table 6, p. 11.

2. William Thomas, Jr., *Nursing Homes and Public Policy* (Ithaca: Cornell University Press, 1969).

3. Thomas, p. 250.

4. Thomas, p. 166.

5. See p. 44 of "Nationwide Survey of State Health Regulations," Levin and Associates, Inc., 1974. Distributed by the National Technical Information Service, U.S. Department of Commerce, Springfield, Va.

The Impacts of Medicaid and Medicare

The Medicare and Medicaid programs enacted in 1965 have often been cited as the explanation for the rapid growth in nursing home utilization that this country has experienced in recent years. In this chapter, we take a close look at the validity of that claim by examining the impact of these programs in such areas as eligibility determination, reimbursement, standards enforcement, and capital expansion.

Medicaid

Eligibility

As far as income eligibility is concerned, Medicaid made a difference only where the criteria under the predecessor OAA or AABD programs were more restrictive—that is, only where nursing home care had been inaccessible to individuals whose income fell above the cash assistance level but below the cost (reimbursement level) of nursing home care. And this would have been the case only where such a state under Medicaid opted to include the medically needy. The only State in the sample that fits this description is Vermont, which did not adopt a medically needy provision until 1968. Such expanded coverage rarely happened in southern states because they already had income eligibility policies in operation under which the "medically needy" were handled so as to be designated programmatically as "categorically needy." Thus, in these southern states, Medicaid brought by and large a simple transfer of coverage of nursing home care from OAA to another funding mechanism with slightly improved federal match, but with essentially no change in income eligibility level.

In those states which had a restrictive income policy in effect and which chose not to include the medically needy under Medicaid, the adoption of Medicaid also obviously had no appreciable effect. As indicated, Medicaid had the greatest impact in those states such as Vermont which previously operated restrictive programs but chose to include a medically needy provision under Medicaid. For other reasons, however, improved access did not seem to result from this in Vermont. Medicaid would have exerted a very significant restrictive impact in those states which operated MAA programs (under which the more liberal income eligibility criteria were extended only to the elderly) but which chose *not* to adopt medically needy provisions. But apparently in every instance (at least this was the case in our sample), states in this situation took very creative and sometimes relatively expensive steps to insure continued nursing home care coverage for those elderly potentially excluded by Medicaid sans a medically needy provision. In West Virginia, such a step took the form of defining skilled care under Medicaid as acute care and funding all long-term care as intermediate care under Title XI. In New Jersey the state continued to cover skilled nursing care for the medically needy but at 100 percent state expense. Obviously, such action was still less costly than adopting a medically needy provision that would have included the nonelderly as well.

All in all, then, except in a very few states, the adoption of Medicaid seems to have had very little effect on the relative access of the population to nursing home care and hence on demand through the raising of income eligibility levels.

As with income eligibility policy, the adoption of Medicaid made a difference with regard to other eligibility criteria only in those states in which these criteria were restrictive before the introduction of Medicaid. In many states limitations on asset levels and on the divestiture of assets, liens on property, postmortem claims, and relative responsibility provisions had been liberalized, left unenforced, or dropped under previous medical assistance programs. In only two of the sample States, Vermont and especially New Jersey, does Medicaid seem to have brought profound changes in these criteria. In Vermont, the removal of the lien provision under Medicaid was cited by respondents as having made a substantial difference in accessibility to nursing home care. This probably would have made a difference under the Medical Assistance for the Aged program as it prohibited liens. However, Vermont's MAA program was not used to fund nursing home care. In New Jersey, the liberalization of limits on assets, the dropping of time limitations on transfer of assets for purposes of obtaining program eligibility, and the removal of the relative responsibility and lien provisions were all pinpointed by respondents as having produced a significant impact on demand for nursing home care there.

In neither State, however, do changes under Medicaid appear to have contributed to a significant rise in the nursing home bed stock over the short run. Perhaps these changes were necessary conditions for the expansion in bed supply which took place in both States several years later; but it is obvious that other conditions are also necessary in order for the impact of eligibility criteria to be felt on growth.

This is not to say that criteria in use for determining eligibility are unimportant, but rather to emphasize that they are only part of the ingredients needed for significant expansion. There could have been a few states in which liberalization of such criteria under Medicaid comprised the key missing ingredient for producing growth, all of the other prerequisite conditions already existing. It appears from our sample, however, that, except in some northern states, or maybe even just northeastern states, significant liberalization occurred prior to the adoption of Medicaid.

Adoption of Medicaid, undoubtedly, was important in at least some states in directly removing some of the stigma traditionally associated with medical assistance programs that had preceded it. This development was helped immensely by the public billing which Medicaid received at the federal level and, in some places, at the state level, as a medical rather than a welfare program. Perhaps of even greater help was the simultaneous passage (and similarity in name) of Medicaid with Medicare, so that Medicaid became indistinguishable from Medicare in the minds of much of the public and consequently picked up Medicare's nonwelfare, "earned benefit" image.

As indicated in the section on eligibility, the Medicaid program has been the impetus behind the states' attempts to tighten up and more systematically structure their medical need assessment procedures. This has come about both as a result of states' desire to save state Medicaid dollars and as a response to HEW requirements. As was pointed out also, however, the states—even those that adopted Medicaid early—have taken serious steps to improve their assessment only since 1970, and some not until the end of the study period.

In some states, Medicaid assessment policies could be contributing to the slowdown in growth which has been typical since the end of this study period. Most likely this has happened, if at all, only in those states which carry out preadmission screening, however. Case study interviews, as well as the results of our phone survey of state officials, reveal that hardly ever is a patient, once admitted to a nursing home, later denied coverage because his condition is judged not to require a further nursing home stay. He or she may be reclassified from skilled to ICF level, but the ICF guidelines are too broad and the alternative living arrangements too narrow once a person has entered a nursing home to result in his or her being denied continued coverage at some level. In this light, preadmission screening seems absolutely necessary if any efforts designed to restrict publicly subsidized care only to those in need of it are to be successful. In only one of our sample States—South Dakota—is there strong indication that medical assessment played a significant role in limited access to nursing home care during any part of the study period, and even there, the influence was indirect.

It is clear that the initial impact of Medicaid was to encourage at the state level the writing of Medicaid assessment regulations and guidelines so as to ensure that virtually everyone would qualify for skilled care, as this was the only level covered by Medicaid. This was the case, that is, in those states not relying on other titles to finance the bulk of their nursing home programs. Since 1972, when ICFs were brought under Medicaid, the principal effect of Medicaid with regard to assessment in many states has been to foster the "rewriting" of state regulations so that most new applicants as well as existing SNF patients are classified as ICF level residents. This has happened, it seems, principally in those states in which reimbursement rates are relatively high. It appears that in those states such as Mississippi, where reimbursement levels are relatively low, nursing home operators are unwilling to accept the ICF rate, thus forcing the state Medicaid office to continue classifying the vast majority of nursing home recipients as SNF level patients.

In conclusion, it is clear that as far as medical assessment eligibility criteria are concerned, Medicaid has exerted at most a negligible impact on demand and hence indirectly on growth of nursing home care during the course of the study period. It has come to affect the level at which care is provided, but seems to have exerted little impact on whether or not an applicant, submitting a certification of care need form signed by his physician, is approved for Medicaid coverage of his or her nursing home care.

Reimbursement

As was the case with eligibility criteria, the adoption of Medicaid made a difference with regard to reimbursement for nursing home care only in those states where those features encouraged or mandated by Medicaid regulations had not been adopted prior to those states' adoption of Medicaid. In those few states still using money payments for nursing home care, Medicaid, of course, brought vendor payments for the first time. In the vast majority of states, however, vendor payments had been initiated under MAA or previous welfare titles. As discussed in chapter 5, adoption of the vendor method of payment may have encouraged nursing home growth; however, determination of independent impact is encumbered by potentially important concurrent developments.

Significantly, higher rates of reimbursement, though not mandated per se by Medicaid legislation or regulations, typically accompanied the states' adoption of the Medicaid program. Rate increases seem to have been a necessary if not sufficient condition for nursing home expansion in many states. Though Medicaid program regulations do not require such rate hikes, the increased federal matching ratios available under Medicaid, as well as the Medicaid guidelines themselves, appear to have encouraged them.

One change in reimbursement policy which Medicaid brought in some states was the introduction of the cost-related reimbursement formula as a replacement for facility-independent rates. This form of reimbursement—required for Extended Care Facilities caring for Medicare patients though, again, not required under Medicaid—apparently was encouraged by HEW communiques to state Medicaid agencies. A few states patterned their programs after the Medicare formula and placed no ceiling on allowable costs. Most states which switched from facility-independent rates to cost-related reimbursement, however, chose sooner or later to impose such a ceiling, so it took only a short time, therefore, before a majority of facilities were reporting costs at or above the ceiling. Because of this development, as well as the presence of other important simultaneous developments affecting nursing homes, it is difficult to assess the impact of this change in reimbursement policy on nursing home growth. The experiences of the sample States in this regard present a mixed picture. (See the section of chapter 5 which discusses the impacts of reimbursement policy on nursing home growth over the study decade.)

The adoption of Medicaid in some states was accompanied by the introduction of uniform rates across counties, state rather than county administered payments, state assumption of the full reimbursement costs, and the end of family supplementation. The effects of these changes in those States which still had the old administrative mechanisms in place when they entered the Medicaid program are extremely difficult to trace. Each one applied only in a relatively few States.

Of these, perhaps the ending of cost-sharing by the counties where this change took place was the most significant because of its potential influence on the reimbursement level which the State set for nursing homes. So long as the counties were responsible for paying a portion of nursing home costs—in some northeastern states this was set at 25 percent—most, it appears, exerted pressure on state legislators and program administrators to keep the rates low so as to minimize county expense. The states, having a much broader and far more flexible tax base as well as the influence of a high level of legislative log-rolling, quite clearly, are typically better able and somewhat more willing to appropriate human service dollars than are most local governments. We were told by one nursing home association director that, in his state, counties which set the nursing home rates and also operated county long-term facilities during the mid-1960s attempted to keep rates low so as to protect the county role as the principal supplier of long-term care. We have no idea how typical this type of organizational enhancement activity was among local jurisdictions contributing to the costs of long-term care, however.

Overall, one would expect rates to be higher on average when only the state is responsible for paying them (although the reverse might be more likely in affluent and politically liberal counties). Level of reimbursement being paid clearly affects the willingness of potential or existing nursing home operators and investors to expand their operations; and, as we have pointed out, increased reimbursement rates appear to have contributed to the growth of the nursing home bed stock experienced over the study period.

Standards

Perhaps through no other mechanism has Medicaid exerted more impact on the nursing home industry than through its influence on standards enforcement. New, more rigorous state licensure standards began to emerge in some states just before Medicaid arrived on the scene; but in almost all states, enforcement of these standards has come through federal efforts to bring nursing homes into compliance with Medicaid (and Medicare) certification standards.

This is not to say, of course, that compliance has been universal or even satisfactory. Ample evidence exists to indicate that many substandard facilities continue to operate. Nevertheless the difference in degree of compliance or enforcement of standards since Medicaid and Medicare arrived is immense.

In some states—for example, Wisconsin—new state licensure standards, enacted in the mid-1960s, for the first time set specific staffing requirements. For most states, however, federal Medicare regulations affecting ECFs, promulgated in 1967, were the first standards imposed on nursing homes which required the presence of a professional nurse in the facility for a specific number of hours per week. It is true that nonprofit nursing homes participating in the Hill-Burton program had to meet highly specific staffing requirements as early as 1954. Such facilities, like ECFs, have never comprised more than a very small percentage of nursing homes, however. Unlike Hill-Burton facilities, though, ECFs could be for-profit operations.

Final Medicaid regulations, applicable to skilled facilities in mid-1970, affected a much larger segment of the nursing home industry. They were patterned after (though not exactly identical to) the Medicare regulations. Medicaid legislation, of course, reflected to a significant degree the Medicare legislation which was enacted simultaneously in 1965. The "medical model," which was followed in developing these standards and which has brought enlarged nursing staffs, nurses' stations, medical charts, pharmacies, and, most recently, medical directors to the nursing home scene, has greatly altered the nursing home image and has made nursing homes more acceptable settings in the minds of those involved in placing patients there. Increased demand stemming from this development, in turn, has helped spur further growth in nursing home care provision.

With the final HEW regulations for SNHs and some federal money made available at that time to the state for carrying out certification processes, including inspections, came also the beginnings of enforcement of the National Fire Protection Association's Life Safety Code. This has turned out to be perhaps the most far-reaching and certainly the most directly visible component in the transformation of the industry. It is true that a fair number of states had been enforcing Hill-Burton standards, which are very similar, to all newly constructed facilities since the mid-1960s or before. Alabama, for example, began in 1959 to require that all new facilities meet such standards before it would issue them an operating license. However, the 1970 Medicaid regulations required for the first time that the Life Safety Code be applied to all nursing homes certified for participation in the program. Although enforcement evolved slowly, this regulation began to result in the replacement of small, older, nonconforming homes with conforming facilities much larger in size. This process has been enhanced further by the application of the Life Safety Code to ICFs in 1974 and the greatly expanded federal funding of inspections and other administrative procedures carried out by the states in certifying facilities for participation as Medicaid providers.

The end result of all this is greatly increased construction costs and, apparently, a subsequent marked reduction in the number of applications submitted to state licensing and planning agencies for the construction of new beds. Thus, this negative effect on growth must be balanced against the increases resulting from the construction of larger facilities in any assessment of net impact of standards enforcement on nursing home growth over the study period. This shrinkage of the potential nursing home investor pool very likely began earlier in those states which required that all new facilities meet Hill-Burton or other expensive standards similar to the Life Safety Code before the code was made applicable to Medicaid-certified facilities in the early 1970s.

Be that as it may, the processes set in motion to ensure that the federal government would get its money's worth in terms of quality care and patient safety out of its financial support of the Medicaid program have produced a large, professionally managed facility which has come at least close to being accepted as a legitimate component of the nation's medical care system.

Capital Funding

Because of the "assurance" of continued, permanent federal subsidization of nursing home care which enactment of Medicaid represented, it appears that the adoption of Medicaid further enhanced the image of the nursing home as a sound financial investment; although, undoubtedly, investor confidence had grown with the adoption of vendor payments under OAA and AABD in the 1950s and with the expansion of federal involvement in nursing home care that came with the MAA program in the early 1960s.[1] Undoubtedly, the promise of Medicaid reimbursement was especially helpful where reimbursements were based on an uncapped reasonable cost formula, thus virtually guaranteeing that nursing homes would not lose money. There were exceptions to this positive role of Medicaid, however. In Florida, respondents informed us that unattractive Medicaid rates and, perhaps more significantly, a series of abrupt changes in reimbursement policy had made it difficult for nursing home investors to obtain funding for construction or expansion activities.

The Hill-Burton program, principally in its role in providing model federal nursing home standards, had a far more long-range effect on the Medicaid program than Medicaid has had on it. The structural standards imposed by the Hill-Burton program on participating facilities, and which some states adopted as licensure requirements for all new constructed facilities in the late 1950s or early 1960s, of course, enormously increased nursing home construction costs and, as a consequence, made large-scale capital funding absolutely essential. Up to that point, nursing homes typically had been converted family dwellings. The imposition of the Life Safety Code under Medicaid for all facilities in the early 1970s, then, greatly broadened the impact of high construction costs, and, consequently, greatly increased the need for sizable capital loans among nursing home providers.

Planning and Investment Controls

Although the evolution of health planning in this country through the Hill-Burton program and then the 1966 Comprehensive Health Planning Act was well underway before the implementation of Medicaid or Medicare, no formal mechanism existed for directly limiting the supply of nursing home beds. This came with the enactment of Section 1122 in the 1972 Social Security Amendments and the requirement for a certificate-of-need program in the 1974 Health Planning and Resources Development Act. (These programs are described in chapter 6.)

Although some might argue that these developments would have come eventually anyway through the sheer evolving dynamics of the health planning idea and the establishment of a planning profession, there is no denying that these recent attempts at health planning and regulation of provider entry, including those for long-term care, grew to a large extent out of the desire of government to control the spiraling costs of health care—especially for acute care services—an increasing proportion of which was being paid for out of Medicaid and Medicare funds.

Section 1122, of course, was tied directly to payment of Medicare and Medicaid monies. Without the impetus of the concern for cost containment, especially in the Medicaid program, it is doubtful that 1122 and certificate of need would have been enacted in the 1970s. These programs, of course, had almost no impact on nursing home growth during the study period because they were just being implemented as the study decade ended. There seems little question, however, that their importance in shaping nursing home expansion is growing and that it will increase as certificate-of-need programs are implemented and become institutionalized in all states.

Conclusion Regarding the Impact of Medicaid

Contrary to what many have assumed, the funding of nursing home care under Medicaid did not set off the rapid growth in nursing home care that has become so visible in the last several years. Rather, by and large, it allowed a continuation under a new funding mechanism of what had existed program-wise since the adoption of vendor payment programs in the 1950s or early 1960s. Similarly, few have realized that the rapid growth which has occurred since the enactment of these programs is a continuation of a pattern of rapid expansion that was even more pronounced in the half decade or so preceding the enactment of Medicaid (see chapter 2). On this basis alone, then, enactment of Medicaid, or Medicare enacted at the same time, for that matter, cannot possibly have played the role of "prime mover" in the expansion of nursing home care that so many have assigned to it.

This is not to say that enactment of Medicaid has had no highly significant localized effects on growth or national long-range impacts on the shape of long-term care provision in this country. Indeed, looking back a decade later, it appears to have revolutionized the nursing home industry in a number of ways. Many of these changes, as we have seen, however, resulted from spin-off regulatory policies—in some instances adopted through regulations patterned after Medicare several years after Medicaid was enacted—rather than directly from its subsidization function.

Medicare

The Social Security Administration began making payments to nursing homes certified as Extended Care Facilities (ECFs) for the care of Medicare beneficiaries requiring skilled nursing services in January 1967. In order to be eligible for Medicare, one had to be age sixty-five or over and eligible for retirement benefits under Title II (eligibility being earned through mandatory contributions to the Social Security trust fund) or under the railroad retirement system. Eligibility for nursing home care was limited to those who met the following requirements: prehospitalization for at least three days, admission within fourteen days of such hospital stay to a certified facility for the same condition which had required hospitalization, and physician's verification of the need for "skilled nursing" in continuation of care. A benefit limitation of 100 days was imposed, but most recipients became ineligible before reaching the maximum through failure to meet Medicare's definition of need for skilled nursing. Medicare covered the full cost of the first twenty days of ECF care; the recipient's coverage was subject to a coinsurance amount (equal to one-eighth of the inpatient hospital deductible) for each succeeding day. The coinsurance amount equaled $5.00 per day in 1967 and $11.50 per day by 1974.

In April 1969, the Bureau of Health Insurance (BHI) added in new regulations the requirement that recipients have "rehabilitation potential," effectively excluding coverage for terminal patients. These regulations also offered a revised and narrowed definition of the term "skilled nursing," which by statute was a precondition to coverage. Under the new definition, which spelled out specifically which medical and nursing services were covered, many patients were denied coverage, and these denials were given retroactive effect. With the passage of the 1972 Amendments to the Social Security Act, the 1969 retrenchment in coverage was liberalized somewhat in the adoption of a policy of "presumptive coverage." Under this policy, beneficiaries upon discharge from a hospital were presumed eligible for ECF care for a set number of days, depending on diagnosis of their condition.

Reimbursement of Extended Care Facilities under Medicare in 1967 began under a reasonable cost formula which placed no upper boundary as such on what those costs could be. Along with a narrowing of eligibility criteria in 1969 came a significantly tighter interpretation of allowable provider costs. The 1972 Amendments left most of the changes in reimbursement policy imposed in 1969 intact but lessened some of the uncertainty of payment by establishing a prospective rather than retrospective basis for disallowance of "unreasonable" costs.

The direct impact of Medicare funding on the nursing home industry has been relatively minor when compared with that of Medicaid. Its importance as a financing mechanism, though significant at first, has shrunk substantially, especially since 1969. Since that point, when Medicare intermediaries began issuing retroactive denials for coverage of care and restricted allowable provider costs, a large-scale withdrawal of nursing homes from participation in Medicare has taken place. Many homes still officially certified under Medicare appear very reluctant to admit Medicare patients. In part as a result, only 5 percent of total federal expenditures on nursing home care were paid for from Medicare funds as of 1976.[2] Even more striking is the fact that, in 1974, only 1 to 2 percent of all nursing home residents were receiving Medicare as the primary source of payment.[3] In that same year, Medicare paid for 8.4 million days of care while Medicaid funded 277 million.[4] Part of the withdrawal of Medicare, undoubtedly, reflects provider backlash from the severe financial straints and disappointments experienced with the program over the period 1969 through 1972—even though, as indicated, since that point these retrenchment policies have been liberalized somewhat. Limited coverage of nursing home care under Medicare—requirements for a preadmission hospital stay of at least three days within the prior two weeks and limitations on days of coverage by principal diagnosis, as well as limits on allowable costs for reimbursement purposes—in effect since the beginning, however, remains and apparently serves to discourage recipient use of and provider participation in the program. Even though by law Medicare reimbursement since 1972 has to be at least equal to, and is often above, the Medicaid rate, this factor does not appear to be attractive enough to compensate for the drawbacks—one of which, we were told by respondents, is the heavy volume of paperwork required under Medicare in order to justify costs.

Those observations notwithstanding, unquestionably some portion of the growth experienced nationwide over the period 1965 to 1969 reflects the influence of Medicare as a financing mechanism. In light of the fact that Medicare and Medicaid legislation were enacted together, it is difficult, of course, to separate out the independent influence of each. The establishment of the Extended Care Facility (ECF) program under Medicare coverage in 1967, with little question, expanded significantly the use of nursing homes for recuperating and postoperative hospital patients. Whereas, before, elderly patients would have had to remain in the hospital until rather fully recovered, transfer to the ECF as soon as the patient no longer requires acute services was made easy by Medicare's continuous coverage of both settings. Of course, the

Social Security Administration extended coverage to nursing homes in order to save Medicare funds as care in a nursing home is substantially less expensive than hospital care. This easy transfer was complicated somewhat after 1969 when, as indicated, Medicare coverage and reimbursement of nursing home care, owing to rapidly increasing utilization, was made more restrictive.

The apparent differential impact of Medicare coverage of nursing home care on nonprofit versus proprietary institutions is worth noting here. Because hospital discharges require placement almost immediately if they are to be covered for nursing home care under Medicare's fourteen-day limitation (between discharge and admission to a skilled nursing home), they almost always have to go into a proprietary facility because most nonprofit facilities have longer waiting lists. Thus, Medicare's share of support in nonprofit homes very likely is considerably less than 5 percent.[5]

It is clear also that the promise of Medicare with its cost reimbursement was in part responsible for the boom in nursing home chain operations and the popularity of nursing home stocks which occurred during that period. Expansionary activity in anticipation of and in reaction to Medicare's promise of reimbursement on an uncapped basis, however, appears to have been spotty—occurring principally in the larger states. No way is available to determine the number of beds built in response to Medicare, but the reports of respondents in the sample States indicate that Medicare's role in stimulating growth was significant in California, Florida, New Jersey, New York, and perhaps South Dakota.

In places like California, the boom in construction which Medicare contributed to in the late 1960s also contributed to the bust in growth when retrenchment in the Medicare program came in 1969. According to respondents, a number of big investors saw a gold mine in Medicare and got into the nursing home business, creating a glut of beds and lowering occupancy rates. Consequently, when the easy money provided by Medicare dried up, they were unable to maintain high profits and thus were forced to sell out. The excess supply of beds accompanied by the rush to unload nursing home operations then contributed, we were told, to a very depressed provider market for the next few years.

As has been the case with Medicaid, the greater importance of Medicare seems to lie more in the role it has played in shaping nursing home care and subsequent growth over the long run than in its short-run impact on nursing home expansion activities. Much of that broader impact, in fact, has come indirectly through the influence of the Medicare program on Medicaid policies implemented in the areas of standards enforcement and reimbursement.

Standards and their enforcement, on the one hand, have made it more costly for potential operators to open up a nursing home. On the other hand—the demand side—these standards have produced a better image for nursing homes among both the public and the medical profession, no doubt leading to increased demand. The response to the costly standards and increased demand has been much larger facilities and, not infrequently, the establishment of corporately owned franchise operations. The net impact of standards may have been an increased bed supply.

Notes

1. See, for example, Betty Reichert, "Humanizing the Institutional Aspects of Long-Term Care," *Human Factors in Long-Term Health Care* (Columbus, Ohio: National Conference on Social Welfare, 1975), p. 64.

2. "Long-Term Care—The Problem That Won't Go Away," *National Journal*, November 5, 1977, pp. 17-27.

3. "Long-Term Care: Actuarial Cost Estimates," Congressional Budget Office Technical Analysis Paper (Washington, D.C.: U.S. Government Printing Office, 1977), p. 48; Jeannine Fox Sutton, "Utilization of Nursing Homes, United States," *Vital and Health Statistics*, Series 13, Number 28, National Center for Health Statistics, U.S. Department of Health, Education and Welfare, 1977, table 2, p. 20.

4. "Long-Term Care: Actuarial Cost Estimates," p. 61.

5. We are grateful to Mr. Benson Rosenberg, Executive Director of the New Jersey Association of Homes for the Aging, for first bringing this differential impact to our attention.

8

Study Conclusions, Policy Implications, and Projections

From the analysis presented in previous chapters, it should be clear that the explanation for dramatic growth in the use of nursing home care between 1964 and 1974 is rather complex and reflects the interactive impacts of a number of rather unique sociohistorical developments as well as governmental policies. Nonetheless, certain variables stand out as particularly important in shaping growth over the study period. In this chapter we attempt to summarize the principal impacts of those key variables. In spite of the rapid growth in this country's nursing home bed stock since the early 1960s, it is also quite clear from our analysis that a state of chronic excess demand for publicly subsidized beds has characterized nursing home care provision throughout the study period. Solutions to the problems created by this bed shortage through specific governmental policies—particularly reimbursement, controls on capital expansion, medical assessment, and funding of alternatives to nursing homes—are also discussed in this chapter.

Conclusion on Determinants of Growth

The enactments of Medicaid and Medicare do not, as many have assumed, mark the beginning of rapid growth in nursing home supply and demand which this country has experienced in the recent past. In terms of average annual percentage increases, growth in number of nursing home beds relative to the size of the elderly population was more rapid before the enactment of Medicaid and Medicare than afterward. The growth that occurred during the early years of the study period appears to have been a continuation of a pattern of rapid expansion which began in the late 1950s and early 1960s.

In many states, those policy changes that allowed the expansion of nursing home care had already been implemented by the time Medicaid and Medicare came along. Medicaid and Medicare, in large measure, functioned to promote further the existing policy trends in long-term care.

Contrary to popular impression, Medicaid appears to have exerted little impact overall on eligibility criteria. By and large, states continued under Medicaid to rely upon the eligibility criteria for nursing home care that they already had in place under their welfare titles. Medicare expanded access from 1967 to 1969, but only for short-term, posthospital care.

Medicaid and Medicare appear to have perpetuated an already expanding supply of nursing home beds through an increased federal match, higher reimbursement rates, and, in some states, a cost-related reimbursement formula. Medicaid and Medicare also seem to have perpetuated an expanding bed supply by further institutionalizing government funding for nursing home care that providers could count on.

The impacts of governmental policies on both demand for and supply of nursing home beds have been significant. They have also been interactive. The impact of reimbursement, for example, was transmitted in part through its effects on other policy areas. In those states which set the nursing home income eligibility level equal to the state's reimbursement rate, for example, the reimbursement level determined to a significant degree the liberality of income criteria and hence the relative accessibility of nursing home care for a large share of the state's impaired elderly population. It appears also that the vigor of state standards enforcement has been affected by the level of reimbursement that the state was paying. Few, if any, states have attempted to enforce standards when the reimbursement rate to nursing homes was clearly inadequate for the providers to profitably comply with the standards. At the same time, however, facilities which met licensure standards in some states were reimbursed at a higher rate than were nonconforming homes.

Not surprisingly, federal encouragement of both demand for and supply of nursing home care has resulted in substantial substitution of nursing homes for care that formerly was provided in more expensive settings—principally mental hospitals and general hospitals.

The impetus behind increased public support for nursing homes seems to have issued in part from the realization that great need for some type of long-term care setting existed among a rapidly growing elderly population. Other sociodemographic developments—for example, accelerated geographical mobility of the population—may have played a role as well.

The Problems of Excess Demand

Government subsidies (given the facility standards imposed) and hence bed supply, nonetheless, have not matched the increased demand stemming from a greatly expanded number of very old elderly, from liberalized eligibility criteria, and from the enhanced attractiveness of nursing home care, owing to the imposition of medically oriented federal standards, as well. Quite obviously, the greatly increased number of very old elderly, who tend to suffer substantially reduced financial resources, has in itself—aside from any liberalization in the eligibility standards—enlarged the number of persons eligible for public support of their care.

This state of chronic excess demand, which appears to have existed throughout the study period, has created some formidable problems for public policymakers in their efforts to provide equal access to long-term care for those who can no longer manage independently. The bed shortage and those problems created or exacerbated by such a shortage may diminish in intensity as the elderly population ages less dramatically over the next decade or two than it has in recent years. On the other hand, recent and emerging government efforts to control supply, owing to rapidly mounting expenditures for nursing home care, could function to perpetuate these problems.

Inappropriate Placement

Except in a few localities, demand for nursing home beds exceeds the supply. Several implications of this situation are fairly obvious but deserve mention. Private-pay patients are selected for admission to nursing homes over Medicaid patients because the private rate is almost always higher; and if the rates are equal, the private-pay residents still require less paperwork. This situation may be especially prevalent in the higher-income states, where more individuals or their families are able to pay the private rates. The problem becomes particularly acute, it appears, in places where total bed supply is controlled through certificate of need. In such locales, caseworkers are extremely hard pressed to find beds for Medicaid recipients. The preferential access accorded private patients wherever this occurs means, of course, that Medicaid patients have to take what is left. That often means the less desirable facilities, and not infrequently, assignment to an inappropriate care level bed—that is, intermediate care rather than skilled, or vice versa. This is not to imply, of course, that private paying patients necessarily are appropriately placed. Their care, however, is not presently a direct public responsibility.

Unlike hospitals, nursing homes under a bed shortage situation appear prone to admit patients with the least serious care needs, given what is classifiable as skilled or intermediate level care. This, of course, makes it especially difficult to place more severely impaired Medicaid recipients. Now that several years of "creaming" have taken place, leaving largely the more seriously impaired in the geriatric wards of the mental hospitals, it appears that those recipients most difficult of all to place often are the discharges from mental hospitals. The end result again is that patients deinstitutionalized from mental hospitals often end up in the very poorest quality homes. Some end up in county nursing homes where care on the whole may be superior, but bed availability in these facilities is extremely limited.

Obviously, a bed shortage situation operates against the improvement of care quality in the poorer facilities. When a state experiences great difficulty in finding beds for Medicaid recipients, it is naturally reluctant to close any existing facilities.

Bed shortages, particularly in areas near state borders, often result in the placement of Medicaid patients in facilities outside of their home state. Such interstate placements, of course, depend on bed availability in adjacent states, relative reimbursement levels of the states involved, and state policy with regard to out-of-state placements. Excess demand also sometimes necessitates the placement of an individual many miles away from his hometown, although within his own state of residence, because that is the only place a bed is available. Besides risking trauma to the individual involved, such action can make visitation of the nursing home resident by relatives and friends extremely difficult.

Ineffectual Needs Assessment

Perhaps in no policy area are the consequences of excess demand more pervasive, even though indirect, than in the area of medical needs assessment. As indicated in chapter 5, overall medical assessment procedures became more formalized over the course of the study period. This came about primarily as a result of federal pressure, especially after 1970.

Final regulations for determining care level designation under Medicaid were published by HEW in September 1975. Up to that point, medical assessment regulations established by the states had been written so that almost everyone in need of some level of nursing or personal care would qualify for whatever level was reimbursed most generously. Prior to inclusion of ICF care under Medicaid in 1972, that was often the skilled level of care. It has continued to be skilled level care wherever, *ceteris paribus,* a large differential between the skilled rate and the intermediate care rate exists or wherever reimbursement rates for both levels are low. It appears that under such circumstances and especially in the context of overall bed shortages, potential providers are uninterested in supplying ICF level care. The implementation of reasonable cost-related reimbursement, effective in 1978, may lessen the arbitrary disparity in rates and thus function to give those who assess medical need for care additional flexibility in their assessment decisions. This outcome could be jeopardized, however, by what portends to be widely varying state interpretations of this requirement.

Under other conditions, assessment teams and physicians may have little else besides ICF beds in which to assign nursing home residents. Some states have decided that virtually all nursing home care shall be designated as ICF level care. In many instances this decision seems to have been forced upon them by the shortage of beds which could meet the Life Safety Code. This policy, in turn, seems to reflect the unwillingness or perceived inability of the state to reimburse nursing homes generously enough to stimulate a larger supply of conforming beds. Under such circumstances, the state may utilize a double standard whereby ICFs are required to meet standards significantly less demanding than those imposed on SNFs. Existing nursing home providers, then, are willing to accept the ICF rate in return for continued certification status as ICFs without having to undergo extensive capital investment.

In spite of more formalized procedures, care need assessors must continue to "stretch" the formal definitions of care need on the basis of constraints imposed by the interface of reimbursement and standards enforcement on bed availability. Until such time as ready availability of beds at all levels becomes a reality, medical assessment and care level placement will remain in large measure an artifact of these exogenous forces rather than a rational procedure.

Meanwhile, effectiveness in eliminating unnecessary care and costs, an objective of the medical assessment process, requires that such assessment be carried out prior to nursing home admission. This is the case because individuals, once admitted to a nursing home, are seldom discharged or assessed at a care need level below that reimbursed by Medicaid. In some instances the nursing home resident, if discharged, has no place to go in the community. Assessment teams also are very sensitive to the traumatic and sometimes fatal effects of change of residence on the frail elderly.

Medical assessment seems likely to remain only marginally effective as a rationing tool in the utilization of long-term care settings also, unless private-pay patients are included in preadmission assessment. A significant proportion of Medicaid supported nursing home residents—for example, one-third in South Dakota—enter nursing homes as private pay patients. Many persons who enter as private patients, whether needing nursing home care or not, soon spend down their assets, especially at the higher prices for care typically charged private pay patients, and then go on Medicaid. As pointed out previously, once they are in a nursing home they are seldom discharged, regardless of the extent of their medical need.

The Role of Planning and Investment Controls

Although this country continues to experience an excess demand for publicly provided nursing home care, it appears that most state legislatures are unwilling to fill all of that unmet demand. They are reluctant to provide additional expansion because of the state cost that would be involved. In addition, it appears that state health planners are beginning to convince state legislative and executive leaders that nursing homes are now used for persons whose care needs could be met more appropriately and less expensively in alternative settings. Many people are inappropriately placed, some planners argue, because supply induces demand—in effect, they say, "Roemer's Law" applies to nursing homes as well as to hospitals.

At first glance, it appears that the most effective way by which the federal government could encourage a movement in the states from a point of excess demand toward a more ample supply would be through easing the cost burden on the states of providing nursing home care—most directly, through a substantially increased federal match under Medicaid. The intended impact of such action, however, might be thwarted in those states that have been moving toward more direct planning controls on bed supply through certificate-of-need programs as well as more indirectly through cost containment measures in the Medicaid program.

For our very limited sample of States with certificate-of-need programs, it appears that enactment tends to stimulate growth initially and then serves to constrain it. Our sample is clearly biased, however, since states included in this study adopted programs before they were required to do so in order to slow the rate of expansion or to control the type of provider entering the nursing home market. States such as Mississippi, which are now adopting programs because they have to, on the other hand, may well follow the pattern of New York and use their authority over provider operating status to allow an expansion of the bed supply for several years before seeking to slow the rate of growth. In those states where such an expansive policy is recognized by providers, an initial growth spurt is less likely to occur, but "healthy" growth for several years could be expected.

Obviously, given an adequate reimbursement level, a certificate-of-need program can be used either to constrain growth or to accommodate market forces. For states desiring to control expansion, a full-fledged certificate-of-need program controlling provider entry through the issuance of operating licenses seems to provide the muscle to do it. In the long run, fiscal limitations very likely will result in widespread use of this mechanism to restrain supply.

The presence of a restrictive certificate-of-need policy in states like New York and California may contribute to the perpetuation of an overwhelming dominance of skilled care beds. With certificate of need, providers apparently feel that they will be "locked in" permanently to whatever level of care they are initially or already providing. Thus, they tend to hold out for the highest certification level designation.

Such constraint on expansion of facilities covered under a state's certificate of need also can lead to rapid growth in those settings not so covered. This seems to have been the case in New York where rapid expansion in "supportive residential facilities" has occurred.[a] With the tight lid on SNF and ICF expansion since 1973, apparently investors and operators sought to get into the business of providing long-term care wherever they could. Many apparently built

---

[a]Supportive Residential Facilities commonly are referred to by such names as boarding homes, sheltered care homes, custodial care homes, adult care homes, personal care homes, and domiciliary care homes. (In New York they are licensed as "Adult Care Homes.") Many residents of these facilities pay for their care from private funds. Many others are supported by public funds, principally SSI, general assistance, and VA. This kind of facility has been around a long time. Although traditionally they have been more closely associated with welfare than with the health arena, they have really fallen between the cracks of public agency responsibility. Nonetheless, this tenuous association with the welfare sphere may act as a countervailing force to pressure for inclusion in the health sphere.

facilities that can be converted to ICFs and SNFs if at any point in the future the lid on their expansion is lifted. This means they built expensive facilities which require a high level of reimbursement to cover capital costs. Economic theory would suggest that expansion of those settings not covered under certificate-of-need regulation is dependent upon the attractiveness of reimbursement to those facilities—that is, the size of the state supplement to the basic SSI payment—relative to standards imposed on them.

Unquestionably, a certificate-of-need program tends to protect existing providers from competition. While it could be used to get rid of operations that provide poor care, it seldom is because of the prevailing shortages of beds and because of the difficulty states encounter in trying to get a nonconforming facility closed.

The likelihood of increased federal funding for nursing home care also may be reduced further as health care planning gains wider and deeper support among large corporations as well as third-party providers. The concern of these interests, of course, is the control of health care costs. Health planners can be expected to increase their influence and success in persuading the public of the rationality of their claims as their profession and visibility grow.

Implications for Federal Action

Much of the rationale for health planning centers around the concern—now widespread at all levels of government, from congressional committees and HEW officials down to the local caseworker—that the long-term setting in which a person receives care be appropriate to his or her care needs and, so far as possible, be congruent with his or her preferences. Thus, there has been growing interest, although as yet limited concrete action, centered on expanding alternatives to nursing home care—principally home care services and supportive residential care facilities.

Coverage of home care services has been extremely limited under Medicare and Medicaid. Although a number of technical and administrative problems exist in the reimbursement arrangements for home health care under Medicare, clearly the most significant limitation on the provision of in-home care services is that such services must be tied to the need for skilled care. Even though the program will reimburse for auxiliary aid services where skilled care is the central component of the care plan, such provision in practice is extremely limited. Medicare does not reimburse for care designed to prevent an acute care episode or institutionalization. Rather, it is limited to use after an acute episode in order to reduce the hospital length of stay. Federal statutory limitations on the use of Medicaid for home care are much less restrictive than for Medicare. Many states, however, have chosen to apply the Medicare limitations to Medicaid as well. Thus, the typical pattern of use of Medicaid for home care at the state level has differed little from that under Medicare.

As a result, the House and Senate aging committees both have conducted a number of hearings on home health care over the past three years. A number of bills designed to expand home care benefits under Medicaid and Medicare or under some other arrangement have also been introduced. HEW held regional hearings on home care in 1976 and is planning to undertake large-scale demonstration projects aimed at determining the costs of home care relative to other long-term settings.

Interviews with State officials in the ten sample States, as well as contacts with local social service administrators and caseworkers involving previous work, strongly suggest that a significant increase in the number of supportive residential facilities is the single most pressing need in long-term care.[1] In those locales with particularly severe shortages of these facilities and supportive community services, individuals and public agencies have been forced to use nursing homes in order to acquire any care at all. As indicated earlier, this results in substantial inappropriate institutionalization in medical facilities and an accompanying drain on Medicaid dollars.

Obviously, the back-up effect of this bottleneck at the supportive residential facility level does not end there. For the inappropriate use of nursing homes for care that could be delivered in less medically intensive settings creates a shortage of nursing home beds. This, in turn, often results either in extended hospitalization for care that could be given in nursing homes were beds available or in discharge directly from a hospital to the patient's home or to a boarding home in cases where nursing care is needed, soon precipitating a return to the hospital. This shortage of licensed community care homes at times has forced individuals and their sponsors, including welfare agencies, to use unlicensed boarding homes, where there may be greater likelihood that medical problems will go unnoticed or untreated until they develop into serious conditions requiring hospital or other medically intense care.

Very recently, congressional attention has turned to problems surrounding the need for and expansion of supportive residential environments. The Keys Amendment, enacted in 1976, mandates state licensing of all those facilities likely to house SSI recipients and removes the prohibition against provision of SSI payments to residents of public group homes of less than sixteen beds. During this past year, the House Aging Committee conducted hearings on the implementation of this legislation. HUD also is currently considering an extension of Section 8 housing allowances to occupants of small community care facilities. Since applicants apparently must be nonproprietary, heavy use of this provision appears unlikely.

Part of the congressional concern centers around what appears to be rapid growth of unlicensed facilities of this type. Whether or not growth in licensed facilities occurs seems to depend upon state standards imposed relative to reimbursement level (presence or size of state SSI supplement), especially as to whether or not the institutional Life Safety Code is applied to these homes. No reliable information for either licensed or unlicensed homes exists, however, to indicate how rapidly the supply is growing, how many persons reside in these facilities, what their needs are, or how well their needs are being met.

All things considered, it seems reasonable to predict that the use of residential care facilities will expand significantly over the next few years, especially if greater public funding for such care becomes available. Such expansion appears even more likely should the emerging restrictive state posture toward expansion of nursing home beds continue. Because of greater complexity of providing home care—for example, the apparent need for informal supports along with formal services to the more severely impaired in order to avoid institutionalization, as well as the need for coordination of formal services and the lack of economies of scale possible in institutional settings—residential care homes might well absorb more of the demand currently expressed for nursing home care than home care services would.

In fact, the proposal to expand home care benefits in order to delay or to prevent institutionalization raises a host of questions which deserve early research attention. How much use of such services would the impaired elderly make? A significant number of elderly individuals are intent on remaining independent as long as humanly possible and thus might resist services, especially if the services are publicly funded and convey a welfare image. A sizable number also might resist the idea of someone coming into their home to carry out household tasks that they are accustomed to doing in their own special manner. To what degree would utilization of home care services vary by socioeconomic status, ethnicity and geographic locale? To what extent would impaired elderly or their families use formal services to supplement care provided informally or to substitute for care provided informally? Available evidence suggests that families are caring for impaired elderly members at home until they are quite ill indeed without benefits of formal services. Thus, would the provision of formal services appreciably lengthen the period of care at home? If it is shown that informal supports are necessary in order for formal services to be effectual, can family surrogates be utilized for those without families? Can the emotive element or the twenty-four-hour availability be duplicated? Physicians are reported to be uninterested in using formal home services for their patients. To what extent would they participate in certifying patients for these services should they become more available? These are some of the questions which make the impact of expanded home care services on demand for nursing home care exceedingly difficult to predict.

Projection of Future Growth of Nursing Home Care

To understand the past can be very satisfying. To predict the future on the basis of that historical knowledge can be much more helpful, though inevitably far more risky. In this section, we discuss those factors which appear most likely to influence the rate of nursing home utilization through 1990.

According to State respondents, growth since the end of the study period

(1974) has been moderate to rapid in only three of the ten sample States—Mississippi, New Jersey, and West Virginia. In another four—California, Florida, New York, and Vermont—growth has been zero or negative, and in the remaining three—Alabama, South Dakota, and Wisconsin—it has been characterized by respondents as slow. From the experience of the sample, then, it appears that growth nationally is proceeding at a much slower rate than that which characterized the study decade. The generalizability of this experience, in fact, is borne out by preliminary National Center for Health Statistics estimates of the national nursing home bed stock as of 1976. The results of the NCHS Master Facility Inventory Census show only a 6 percent growth in absolute number of beds since 1973—from 1,107,358 to 1,173,519. (Between 1969 and 1971 and then between 1971 and 1973, the equivalent rates were 30 and 21 percent, respectively.) As we shall see, it seems likely that this recent trend will turn out to be part of a long-range pattern rather than a short-term deviation.

It appears that the supply of nursing home beds expands only when developments take place which increase private demand or which enhance the profitability of providing care for Medicaid recipients. Medicaid profitability is a manipulable factor determined in large measure by federal and state actions with regard to reimbursement rates. Recently, federal policy has enhanced the potential profitability of caring for Medicaid recipients through the requirement that states establish cost-related reimbursement formulas. This is scheduled to take effect in 1978. As noted before, enhanced profitability as a consequence of this federal action is only potential because of the apparent wide latitude allowed states in the development of reimbursement formulas. It is likely that this potential will be realized in some states but not in others.

States are likely to act to increase the bed supply in order to fill the unmet need only if demand pressure intensifies or if they come to view nursing homes as a desirable substitute for other care settings—for example, mental hospitals or institutions for the mentally retarded. Again, demand pressure can be expected to lessen somewhat as a result of a reduced rate of increase in the size of the frail elderly population. At the same time, it would be wise to recognize the possibility that such lessened pressure could be partially offset by such historical developments as the very substantial reduction in the fertility rates of women of child-bearing age during the Depression era. Many of these women will be entering the ranks of the older elderly during the 1980s with significantly lessened chances of having an adult child who can provide assistance that might allow them to postpone admission to a nursing home.

Some increase in demand for nursing home care from the nonelderly disabled population can be expected. This development springs in part from policies adopted under such program as Vocational Rehabilitation which stress use of similar benefits, such as Medicaid, whenever possible to accomplish rehabilitation. According to Congressional Budget Office estimates, the total pool of nonaged disabled needing nursing home care is small (140,000 nationally in 1975), so that impact of demand from this segment of the population would be minor. Some increased demand from the younger population as well as the older population may come from intensifying efforts of all third-party payers to reduce lengths of stay in acute care hospitals. The success of these efforts is less than certain, however, because of the limited coverage of nursing home care provided by Medicare and private insurers.

The growing effort to transfer the developmentally disabled out of large state institutions into nursing homes certified under Medicaid as ICF-MRs obviously will add to the size of the total nursing home population. It appears that expansion of these specialized nursing homes is just beginning to take off. Relatively rapid growth in the next few years can be expected, although some states are seeking to control closely both the size and location of these facilities.

Deinstitutionalization efforts aimed at substituting nursing homes for care of mental hospital patients, on the other hand, appear to be waning. It appears that the "creaming" process has left largely a relatively small number of more seriously impaired patients who are much more difficult to place. Moreover, practitioners are now having second thoughts about the wisdom of substituting nursing home care for treatment in mental hospitals. Perhaps most significantly, the Supplemental Security Income program implemented in 1974 apparently has encouraged heavy use of boarding homes and the like for former and would-be mental hospital patients.[2]

On balance, it appears very unlikely that, in the face of budgetary concerns, many states will take the initiative to expand the nursing home bed supply. In a growing number of states, nursing home expenditures are exceeding those for all other Medicaid services. Already a number of states are seeking to restrict eligibility and are considering ways by which relative responsibility, family supplementation, and restrictions against transfer of assets might be reimposed. States and now the Congress also are "threatening" other steps unpopular with providers to contain Medicaid costs—for example, requiring facilities to be certified for Medicare or for ICF level care in order to retain certification as a Medicaid certified SNF.

A number of states also are actively seeking to expand the availability and use of alternatives to nursing homes, principally supportive residential facilities— adult foster homes, sheltered care homes, custodial care homes, and the like—in large part to reduce costs, but also to obtain a fuller continuum of care modes so that needs might be better matched with care settings. As a result of emerging interest at both the state and federal levels in greater use of these community care settings, enhanced funding for these settings may be expected. Many states would also like to expand home care in order to reduce dependence on nursing homes. This will happen, it appears, only if federal coverage of such care is expanded significantly under modified Medicare and Medicaid programs, National Health Insurance, or some other funding mechanism.

States may also use investment controls in order to hold down nursing bed supply, and hence costs. As indicated, use of certificate-of-need programs to control nursing home expansion is increasing. If, as expected, reimbursement becomes less state manipulable, investment controls can be expected to gain dramatically in importance as the chief means states possess for shaping the nursing bed supply.

In fact, a number of amendments to the 1974 National Health Planning and Resources Development Act (which contains direct investment controls authorization) currently being considered in Congress, if enacted, could lead to a substitution among long-term care settings opposite in direction from that which contributed to the growth of the nursing home industry. These bills are aimed at encouraging the states to convert the growing number of unused general hospital beds to use for long-term care patients rather than expand the nursing home bed supply.[3] The enactment of any of these proposed amendments, of course, would produce an additional, and potentially very significant, depressing effect on further nursing home growth, at least in some locales.

All factors considered, it appears that the most dramatic growth of the nursing home industry is past and that future expansion will proceed at a significantly reduced rate. Slower growth of the older elderly population and governmental efforts to expand use of alternatives—principally supportive residential facilities—which potentially would function to drain off some of the chronic unmet need, can be expected to contribute the most to less intense demand. At the same time, however, government policies aimed at controlling Medicaid costs, including controls on provider entry, may well discourage supply.

Notes

1. See Burton Dunlop, "An Informal Look at the Long-Term Care Placement Decision Process in a Metropolitan Area," Working Paper 975-10 (Washington, D.C.: The Urban Institute, 1975).

2. See, for example, U.S. Senate, "The Role of Nursing Homes in Caring for Discharged Mental Patients," Supporting Paper No. 7, Subcommittee on Long-Term Care, Special Committee on Aging (Washington, D.C.: U.S. Government Printing Office, 1976).

3. See *Long-Term Care,* Volume 7, Number 11, March 17, 1978, newsletter (Washington, D.C.: McGraw-Hill, Inc.), p. 2.

Appendix A:
A Synoptic History of
the Nursing Home

We can trace at least three paths of origin of today's nursing home.[1] One is the local almshouse or county poor farm. The second is the private home for the aged first established by charitable organizations just before the turn of the century to provide shelter and maintenance for the well elderly who were often of limited financial means or bereft of family. The third is the private proprietary boarding home which emerged about the same time as the home for the aged but which catered to those able to pay for the supervision and personal care that such homes offered.

As the need for nursing care arose among the residents of the homes for the aged and boarding homes, many of these facilities added nursing staff and gradually evolved into nursing homes or personal care homes with infirmaries. The real boost to these two settings, however, came with passage of the Social Security Act of 1935. With its OASI and OAA provisions, the act both greatly expanded the number of persons able to purchase boarding home or nursing home care and allowed elderly persons to live by themselves.

This latter development in itself appears to have helped to transform in a relatively short time many boarding homes and homes for the aged into nursing homes, because elderly persons with incomes from Social Security programs with which to maintain themselves waited until they needed nursing care before entering one of these facilities. Some boarding homes also apparently added nursing care in order to gain a competitive edge over other boarding homes. The prohibition against payment of Social Security benefits to residents of public homes—almshouses and the like—until passage of the 1950 Amendment to the Social Security Act further encouraged the expanded use of private boarding homes, homes for the aged, and nursing homes. In fact, this statutory prohibition caused a substantial diminution in the use of public facilities until they too emerged as full-fledged nursing homes with greatly expanded medical staffs after 1950. The metamorphosis of county or city facilities often included a stage as a chronic disease hospital and, in fact, many public nursing homes are parts of county hospital complexes. The role of county facilities as the care setting of last resort for the down-and-outer type has remained unaltered, however. Today, they typically serve not only the poorest but also some of the sickest nursing home patients.

The dramatic switch from predominance of long-term care delivered in boarding homes to that provided in nursing homes is indicated in census statistics for years 1940 through 1960. These show that the proportion of all institutionalized elderly who resided in "group quarters" declined from 41 percent in 1940 to 12 percent in 1970, while the proportion residing in nursing homes increased from 34 to 72 percent of all institutionalized persons over the same period.[2]

By the 1930s and 1940s, however, there were still precious few nursing homes delivering anything more than the bare minimum of nursing supervision. As a result, in part, general hospitals were used rather extensively for persons with chronic illnesses.

Bed shortages became a severe problem because the demand for acute care was increasing dramatically as a result of greatly expanded insurance coverage. By the 1950s hospitals were fast becoming far more specialized as centers for the treatment of acute illness—a development much encouraged by the medical profession as well as Blue Cross and other medical insurers—and were seeking ways to empty their beds of patients with chronic illnesses in order to make room for acute cases. By the late 1950s, they had begun to look to nursing homes for the care of the chronically ill. Congress actively encouraged this substitution by extending the Hill-Burton program to nursing homes in 1954 and through coverage of nursing home care under several Social Security titles: Old Age Assistance, Aid to the Aged, Blind and Disabled, Medical Assistance for the Aged, and then later, Medicaid and Medicare.

Since the early 1960s nursing homes clearly have emerged as *the* specialized setting for the delivery of long-term care for the elderly in this country. Virtually no one questioned the medical model employed for their development both by Congress and the Public Health Service. The operation of that model is easily discernible, first in the standards applied to Hill-Burton facilities as early as 1954, and then in those applied to all Medicare and Medicaid certified homes. With these, nursing homes were made equivalent to skilled homes.[3] The imposition of these standards, of course, significantly increased demand and costs and contributed to the use of skilled facilities for care that from a medical standpoint, at least, could be met in a less care intensive environment.

Made aware of these developments, Congress set up the ICF program first under Title XI in 1967 and then brought it under Medicaid funding in 1972. Now the Congress is beginning to turn its attention to expansion of home care and residential care facilities, because it is widely believed that nursing homes, even of the ICF ilk, are too intensive and too expensive for the provision of the kind of residential and personal care needed by many elderly individuals—the type of care formerly provided by boarding homes and homes for the aged before so many evolved into nursing homes.

The search for alternatives to nursing homes is intensified today by the further evolution of utilization review in hospitals and resultant heavier use of nursing homes for more and more patients who formerly would have been cared for in hospitals. This review process, carried out by both public and private third-party payers—as well as the funding of posthospital nursing home care through Medicare, of course—is producing a nursing home population, especially at the skilled level, of sicker patients, further perpetuating the medical care role of the nursing home. In effect, the nursing home, at least the skilled facility unit, is becoming a specialized setting for the subacute, recuperative, and rehabilitative patient, while the resident needing largely personal care or protective oversight is less often seen there, and increasingly, it appears, will be cared for in other settings.

Notes

1. For a detailed history of nursing homes, see: Robert Moroney and Norman Kurtz, "The Evolution of Long-Term Care Institutions," in S. Sherwood, ed., *Long-Term Care: A Handbook for Researchers, Planners and Providers* (New York: Spectrum Publications, 1975), and accompanying references; William C. Thomas, Jr., *Nursing Homes and Public Policy* (Ithaca: Cornell University Press, 1969); R. Markus, "Nursing Homes and the Congress," Congressional Research Service, Library of Congress, November 1, 1972; "The Availability and Financing of Nursing Home Care," *Blue Cross Reports,* April-June 1964; Helen McGuire, "New Laws and Regulations Must Focus on Continuity of Care," *Hospitals,* October 16, 1975, pp. 63-67; Barbara Manard et al., *Old Age Institutions* (Lexington, Mass.: Lexington Books, D.C. Heath and Company, 1975); Christopher J. Crocker, "A Brief History of Old Age Institutions in the United States," mimeographed (Charlottsville, Va.: University of Virginia Center for Program Effectiveness, 1974).

2. See Manard, p. 126.

3. The Public Health Service not only established standards that were medically oriented, but actively encouraged the construction of facilities that were hospital-based. Of those facilities participating in the Hill-Burton program that were not hospital-based, the Service assured that they would be integrated into the medical care system by requiring that they negotiate formal agreements with hospitals for ready transfer of patients and the sharing of equipment and staff. In fact, the Service's Division of Chronic Diseases initiated studies in 1960 to learn how such agreements could best be facilitated. It is quite clear also that the Senate Finance Committee, which has exercised final jurisdiction in Medicaid/Medicare matters, has viewed quality care synonymously with medical care.

Appendix B: Characteristics of Federal Programs Affecting the Provision of Nursing Home Care: 1950-1974

Introduction

In the following pages, characteristics of the major federal and federal/state programs which had a direct impact on the supply of and demand for nursing home care during the period 1950 to 1974 are outlined. Programs discussed are of two types—federal subsidies of the cost of construction, expansion and/or modernization of nursing homes, and federal contributions to the cost of purchasing nursing home care. Attention is focused on those aspects of each program having a direct bearing on the provision of nursing home care. Sources used in compiling this section were primary sources (for example, pieces of legislation, federal regulations), federal documents on medical assistance programs, general works in the area of federal provision of medical care, and extensive interviews with current and former federal and state officials. An attempt has been made to cite relevant primary sources; see the bibliography for a list of other sources consulted in the preparation of each section.

Federal Capital Subsidies

Through the three programs described below, the federal government responded to a perceived shortage of nursing home beds in the 1950s and 1960s with grants, loans, and loan guarantees for the construction of nursing homes.

Hill-Burton Program

The Hospital Survey and Construction Act of 1946, or Hill-Burton Program, as it is more popularly known, authorized grants to states for (1) surveying needs and developing state plans for the construction of hospitals and public health centers and (2) assisting in constructing and equipping needed public and voluntary nonprofit general, mental, tuberculosis, and chronic disease hospitals, and public health centers. In 1954 the Hill-Burton law was amended to provide federal financial support for the construction of nonprofit nursing homes and other types of nonproprietary long-term care institutions.

Only facilities capable of providing "skilled nursing care" were to be eligible for federal financial assistance under the new program. Such care was defined to include "nursing services and procedures employed in caring for the sick which require technical skill beyond that which an untrained person possesses." The law also required that the nursing care and other medical services provided by any Hill-Burton-financed nursing home be "prescribed by, or . . . performed under the general direction of, persons licensed to practice medicine or surgery in the state." The term "nursing home" was defined as a "facility for the accommodation of convalescents or other persons who are not acutely ill and not in need of hospital care, but who require skilled nursing care and related services. . . ."

The Community Health Services and Facilities Act of 1961 increased appropriation authorization for construction of nursing homes from $10 million to $20 million annually. And in 1964 the Hospital and Medical Facilities Amendments authorized $350 million for new construction, modernization, and replacement of long-term care facilities over a five-year period. This category combined the previously separate grant programs for chronic disease hospitals and nursing homes; the annual ceiling was raised from $40 million to $70 million.

Amendments in 1968, 1970, and 1973 extended the Hospital and Medical Facilities Survey Construction program through June 1974. The 1970 Medical Facilities Construction Amendments also authorized the program to provide direct loans and loan guarantees with interest subsidies in addition to grants. Grants for the construction and modernization of long-term care facilities were authorized at the level of $85 million annually for 1971-1973 and at $20.8 million for 1974.

Small Business Administration Loan Program

In testimony on the 1954 Hill-Burton Act amendments, witnesses for the American Nursing Home Association pointed out that private, as well as public, sources of construction and improvement capital for proprietary nursing homes were virtually nonexistent. Two federal programs were implemented in the late 1950s in response to this need. The first, the Small Business Administration loan program for proprietary nursing homes, was inaugurated in 1956. To be eligible for SBA loan assistance, a nursing home operation had to qualify as a "small business," meaning that its annual volume of receipts could not exceed $1 million. Loans were available to convalescent and nursing homes for new construction, expansion, equipment and supplies, and for working capital. The amount of a loan could not exceed $350,000 and carried a maximum interest rate of 5.5 percent over a term of ten years. SBA loan outlays averaged $6.9 million per year for the period FY 1969-1974. The outlays in FY 1972 and FY 1973 were $2.7 million and $1.7 million respectively. Besides making direct loans, the SBA also guaranteed commercial loans to qualifying businesses. The value of SBA loan guarantee commitments was $12 million in FY 1972 and $9 million in FY 1973.

Federal Housing Administration Mortgage Insurance Program

Far more significant in terms of the number of facilities funded than the SBA loan program was the mortgage insurance program for proprietary nursing homes established by Congress in Section 232 of the Housing Act of 1959. Under this program, the FHA insured lenders against loss on mortgages for the construction and rehabilitation of long-term care facilities. As a source of capital, the FHA loan program was more attractive to nursing home operators than the SBA program in two respects: the maximum term on loans was twenty years rather than ten as under the SBA program (this FHA maximum was later increased to forty years), and the ceiling on mortgage principal was $12.5 million or 75 percent of the estimated value of the project to be financed (later increased to 90 percent), rather than $350,000 as under the SBA program. The maximum interest rate was originally set at 6 percent of the outstanding principal balance (exclusive of the premium charges for mortgage insurance) but was adjusted upward periodically so as to remain in line with or slightly below prevailing interest rates. One condition of FHA as well as SBA loan insurance was proof in the form of a certificate of need from the appropriate state agency that a need existed for the proposed beds.

The value of FHA-insured loans for construction of long-term care facilities averaged $95 million per year for the period FY 1969-1974. The value of insured loans for FY 1973 and FY 1974 was $84 million and $82 million, respectively. By 1974, 110,485 nursing home beds had been constructed with the help of Section 232 loans.

Federal Participation in the Purchase of Nursing Home Care

Federal participation in the direct purchase of nursing home care began in 1950 with the authorization of vendor payments (payments made directly to medical care providers) under the federal/state welfare program, Old Age Assistance. In some states, Old Age Assistance, Aid to the Blind, and Aid to the Disabled were collapsed into a single program, Aid to the Aged, Blind and Disabled (AABD). Federal policy with respect to OAA and AABD coverage of nursing home care was identical. As in succeeding federal/state medical assistance programs, state participation in the vendor payment program was optional. Beginning in 1956, federal matching funds available for medical vendor payments were no longer limited by monthly dollar ceiling amounts per *individual* recipient. In other words, the amount of federal matching was determined by the average of all payments rather than by a maximum related to each individual payment. This change enabled states to receive federal participation for larger medical expenses (for example, nursing home care) in individual cases.

The passage of the Kerr-Mills Bill in 1960 affected categorical assistance for the aged in two ways: (1) by providing special incentive federal matching for medical vendor payments in behalf of OAA recipients; and (2) by creating a new program of vendor payments called Medical Assistance for the Aged (MAA, also known as Kerr-Mills), under which vendor payments would be made in behalf of the "medically needy" elderly (those too poor to be able to meet their medical expenses, but with incomes too high to enable them to qualify for OAA).

With the adoption of Title XIX in 1965, states were given the option of replacing their medical vendor payment programs under the welfare titles with a Medicaid program. Federal participation in vendor payments under the welfare titles continued in non-Medicaid states until January 1, 1970. By that date all states except Alaska and Arizona had adopted Medicaid programs.

Medicare, the fourth program through which federal funds were used to purchase nursing home care, was, unlike the other three, entirely federal and thus did not vary significantly across states. In characterizing these four programs, only those aspects of the program which affected the provision of nursing home care are discussed. While primary attention is focused on federal policies and provisions, typical state policies are described whenever possible.

Old Age Assistance

Levels of Nursing Homes Covered. Federal regulations had required since 1953, that states license all nursing homes receiving federal public assistance dollars, but left to the discretion of the states what levels of care would be paid for by OAA. Most states covered a wide variety of care levels, reimbursing vendors for "nursing home" care in facilities ranging from rooming houses to facilities providing skilled care.

General Eligibility. Eligibility criteria were set by each state; the federal government intervened only in prohibiting age requirements of more than sixty-five years and overly restrictive residence requirements.[1] States determined financial eligibility through the application of means tests. A state would establish a "standard of assistance" (in some states a fixed dollar figure and in others a figure which varied somewhat depending on the recipient's budget) considered to be the minimum amount of income sufficient for subsistence; states fell into three categories on the basis of how the standard of assistance was applied. "In-or-out" states deemed individuals whose incomes fell below this basic need level financially eligible for both money payments and medical vendor payments; individuals whose incomes fell above the standard of assistance were deemed ineligible regardless of their ability to meet the cost of care. Other states modified this approach somewhat, allowing the cost of nursing home care to be included in certain applicants' budgets, thus enabling them to qualify for money and vendor payments (if the state had a vendor payment program). In the third group of states, individuals whose incomes fell above the standard of assistance were ineligible for money payments but were entitled to "spend down" into eligibility for vendor payments. These individuals, classified as "vendor payment only" or "medical care only" cases, were entitled to a state contribution toward the difference between their medical costs and incomes.

Eligibility for Nursing Home Care. Any individual otherwise eligible for OAA (meeting age and residence requirements and so on) whose income fell below the standard of assistance in his state was eligible for any nursing home benefits offered by the state. These benefits took the form of direct money payments to the recipient which he paid to the nursing home for his care, or vendor payments to the nursing home, or some combination of money and vendor payments. The recipient's income was applied to the cost of his care. Most states set a maximum on the amount which they would contribute toward an individual's nursing home costs, although this maximum was often higher than the general OAA payment maximum. In some states nursing homes were required to accept the state's reimbursement as full payment, while in others, homes were permitted to charge the recipient and/or his family a limited supplemental amount. For example, in 1964, Florida would make a vendor payment of up to $100 in behalf of a recipient, but only to a nursing home which charged the recipient at a rate of no more than $300 per month. In other words, the vendor payment maximum was $100 and the maximum rate which could be charged was $300. Typically, this maximum recognized charge was also the maximum amount which could be included in an applicant's budget for nursing home care. In Florida, for example, an applicant was considered financially eligible for OAA assistance if his income (minus a $10 per month personal incidentals allowance) was less than the monthly cost of care or $300, whichever was lower. With the exception of a few other states (for example, Colorado), only southern states permitted family supplementation, a practice which enabled these relatively poorer states to provide more expansive nursing home coverage than they would have otherwise been able to afford.

In a state with a "medical care only" provision, an individual whose income fell above the cash assistance level but below the cost of nursing home care was eligible for assistance from OAA if that program included nursing home services among the benefits available to its "medical care only" cases. The OAA assistance usually took the form of vendor payments to the nursing home. In some states these vendor payments were only for medical care; the recipient was expected to use his income to cover his maintenance costs (room and board and personal care costs for a nursing home resident). Payments in behalf of "medical care only" cases were also subject to maximums. A recipient was not guaranteed the full amount he needed to meet the cost of nursing home care. For example, an individual with a monthly income of $150 needing nursing home care costing $300 per month might receive vendor payments in the amount of $75 from OAA. He would be expected to obtain the $75 per month difference through what was called "mobilization of community resources," an appeal to charities, relatives, county assistance programs, and so on. If unable to come up with the full amount required to pay for the needed level of care, an individual was faced with several unattractive options: settling for a lower, cheaper level of nursing home care; locating a nursing home (often in another part of the state) which would provide him with the services he required at a price he could afford; entering a public institution including a mental health hospital; or foregoing any formal care provision.

Reimbursement Policy. Reimbursement policy was state determined and varied considerably across the states. The most common policy was to reimburse on a flat-rate basis, paying a single flat rate statewide, several flat rates for different levels of care, or flat rates negotiated at the county level.

Federal/State Cost Sharing Arrangements. The federal government paid 80 percent of the first $30 (in either money or vendor payments) per OAA recipient plus between 50 and 65 percent (the exact amount being determined by a comparison of the state's per capita income with that of the United States—the poorer the state, the larger the federal share) of the next $35 (in either money or vendor payments), *and* between 50 and 80 percent of the amount over $65 spent by the state on medical payments up to an average of $12 per recipient.[2] Thus, the maximum amount subject to federal participation was $65 multiplied by the number of recipients plus that amount above the $65 average for all recipients which was expended for vendor medical payments up to an average of $12 per recipient. The addition of this $12 medical payment allowance encouraged states to make vendor payments in behalf of recipients since, while only the first $65 in money payments per recipient was subject to federal matching, an additional $12 would be matched by the federal government if it was made in the form of vendor payments.

Thus, a state received federal matching of 80 percent of its expenditures if it spent a per recipient average of $30 or less in either money or vendor payments. It received federal matching of between 65 and 80 percent of its expenditures if it spent a per-recipient average of between $30 and $65 in either money or vendor payments. It received no federal matching for expenditures over $65 unless the expenditures were in the form of vendor payments, in which case the state received federal matching of between 50 and 80 percent on the amount spent up to a maximum of $12 per recipient. In 1961 the per-recipient vendor payment addition was increased to $15.

The financial incentive to create vendor payment programs was effective. In June 1960 (the earliest year for which complete data are available), twenty-nine of the fifty-one OAA programs (the fifty states and the District of Columbia) paid for nursing home care through money payments, fourteen through vendor payments and eight through some combination of money and vendor payments. One year later, eight additional states were purchasing nursing home care through vendor payments, and by 1964 all but eleven states used vendor payments to cover at least part of the cost of nursing home care for OAA recipients.

Standards. The federal government played no role in standard-setting except to require (beginning in 1953) that there be a state standard-setting authority responsible for establishing and maintaining standards for nursing homes and other medical care institutions and, in 1960, to define a "medical institution" for the purposes of participation of such institutions in public assistance programs.

Medical Assistance for the Aged

With the passage of the Kerr-Mills Bill in 1960, states were given the option of participating in this federal/state vendor payment program which theoretically helped finance the medical care of elderly individuals whose incomes fell between the OAA cash assistance level and the cost of needed medical services. Of the nineteen states which had adopted MAA programs by October 1962, seven included long-term nursing home care as a benefit, and six, short-term care. By January 1966, forty-three states and the District of Columbia were participating in the MAA program; twenty-three covered some sort of long-term nursing home care; nine more covered short-term nursing home stays.

Levels of Care Covered. All state MAA plans were required to provide for the inclusion of "some institutional and some non-institutional care and services." The federal enabling legislation suggested that skilled nursing home care be included among the institutional services.[3] Most, but not all, states chose to include some sort of nursing home care in their MAA programs, but in a number of states the maximum reimbursement rate was too low to pay for much more than personal care.

General Eligibility. Eligibility was state determined with the exception of the following federal requirements: no age requirements of more than sixty-five years could be imposed; no residence requirement which would exclude any individual residing in the state could be imposed; no enrollment fee, premium, or similar charge could be imposed as a condition of any individual's eligibility; and recipients were to be individuals who were not recipients of OAA but whose income and resources were insufficient to meet the costs of medical care.[4]

States were authorized to determine financial eligibility; the methods of eligibility determination used fell into two general patterns. "In-or-out states" set a basic amount for income and assets so that all persons with less than that maximum were eligible for MAA in relation to their medical care needs. Persons with more income than the maximum were ineligible for any benefits. MAA eligibility determination in these states differed from OAA eligibility determination only in that the cut-off level was, in theory, at least, higher. Other states set a basic amount deemed necessary for self-maintenance of the applicant and his dependents that was to be *excluded* from consideration as available to meet costs of medical care; all income and assets in excess of this protected amount were considered available to meet the costs of medical care. This system, unlike the first, made eligibility rest on an applicant's ability to meet his medical costs (in effect, the eligibility level was equal to the sum of an individual's self-maintenance costs and his medical costs).

Thus, in an "in-or-out state" any individual otherwise eligible whose income fell below the eligibility level was eligible for MAA vendor payments; an individual whose income fell above the level was ineligible regardless of his ability to meet his medical costs. In a state which determined eligibility through the second system, an individual was eligible if his income was less than the sum of his medical costs and the amount deemed necessary for his maintenance.

Eligibility for Nursing Home Care. An individual in an "in-or-out state" whose income fell below the standard of assistance was entitled to vendor payments for nursing home care if such care was among the medical services covered by his state's MAA program and if he met other eligibility criteria (for example, limits on assets, residence, and age requirements). Of course, states also required applicants for nursing home vendor payments to meet conditions establishing medical need for such services. For example, a state might specify that payments would be made only for care immediately following discharge from a hospital or upon a physician's recommendation.

Determination of eligibility for nursing home care in states which set the financial eligibility level at the sum of self-maintenance costs and medical costs differed from determination of eligibility for noninstitutional services. Either the medical and maintenance costs of nursing home care had to be separated or a special (much lower) protected maintenance amount had to be established for determining the financial eligibility of residents of nursing homes. Both of these options were used by states.

Although in theory the MAA program was to provide vendor payments to those individuals whose incomes disqualified them for OAA, some states, like New York, provided nursing home care to individuals whose incomes fell below the OAA cash assistance level through MAA instead of OAA. On the other hand, although financial eligibility criteria under MAA were intended to be less restrictive than those under OAA, in 1963 it was found that in fourteen states the MAA income levels were more rigidly interpreted and often lower than those for OAA.

Relative Responsibility and Liens. The Kerr-Mills Bill did not prohibit family or relative responsibility provisions; in 1963, twelve of the twenty-eight states participating in the MAA program required an applicant's relatives to be subjected to means tests. However, states differed substantially in how rigorously this provision was enforced. While some "relative responsibility" states (for example, New Jersey), denied coverage to an applicant if the financial accounts of relatives showed them to be capable of caring for the applicant, others (for example, Florida) merely inquired whether a child who was currently contributing to the applicant's income chose to continue to do so.

The Kerr-Mills legislation prohibited states from placing a lien on a recipient's property prior to his death, one onerous consequence of accepting OAA assistance in many states. Nine states did require a MAA recipient to give the state the right to collect from his estate (or that of his spouse) after death by means of postmortem claims; however, these states rarely exercised this prerogative.

Reimbursement Policy. The federal MAA legislation did not specify any reimbursement policy; the practice most commonly followed by the states was to pay on a "reasonable cost" basis up to a maximum rate. This ceiling was low enough in most states to serve as a de facto flat rate.

Federal/State Cost-Sharing Arrangements. The federal government agreed to pay from 50 to 80 percent of the cost of vendor payments (the exact percentage to be determined by a comparison of the state's per capita income with that of the United States as a whole—the poorer the state, the larger the federal share.[5] The structure was one of open-ended federal cost-sharing, without limitations on individual payments or on total state expenditures; cost control was left to the states. In the case of nursing home care, states controlled costs by imposing rigid financial eligibility criteria, paying low reimbursement rates and thus restricting bed supply and/or limiting the nursing home benefit to short-term or posthospital care.

Standards. As under OAA, the federal government played no role in setting or enforcing standards for nursing homes receiving MAA vendor payments except that these institutions were subject, at least theoretically, to inspections from federally mandated state standard-setting authorities.

Medicaid

Title XIX, or Medicaid, was signed into law in July 1965. This state-option medical assistance vendor payment program began paying for nursing home care in participating states in January 1966. Medicaid replaced the vendor payment programs of the categorical assistance titles; when a state began making payments through Medicaid, it lost federal participation in MAA and in vendor payments (but not money payments) under OAA. States which chose not to participate in Medicaid continued to receive federal matching funds for OAA and MAA until January 1970, when federal sharing of vendor payment under the categorical assistance programs ended in all states.

The two levels of nursing home care eventually paid for by Medicaid are discussed separately below.

Skilled Care. One of the five basic services required of all state Medicaid programs was skilled nursing home services for persons twenty-one years and older (care in a tuberculosis or mental hospital was not to be covered). No definition of "skilled nursing home" existed until the publication in June 1966 of Supplement D to the Handbook of Public Assistance.

General Eligibility All states participating in the Medicaid program were required to extend eligibility to all recipients of money payments under OAA, AB, APTD, AABD, or AFDC. The recipients in this group were known as the "categorically needy." A second group of recipients whose coverage by states was required included those who would be eligible for money payments under one of the five categorical assistance programs were it not for a specific state provision overridden by Title XIX. The two such provisions affecting eligibility of the elderly were durational residence requirements and age requirements in excess of sixty-five years.

Besides these two groups whom states were required to cover, there were specified groups whose inclusion was at the option of the state, and for whom federal cost-sharing was available. States could, of course, also include whomever else they pleased, but no federal matching money was available. The first of these optional groups together with the second of the mandatory groups described above made up the "categorically related" group. In this group were those individuals who would be eligible for money payments under a categorical assistance program if the state's program were as liberal as permitted by federal regulations—for example, individuals who would be eligible for AFDC-UP except for the fact that their state had no such program. A second group whose coverage was at the option of the state was the "noncategorically related medically needy." The one group of elderly affected by this option consisted of those individuals who met the "essential person" definition. Under this option, a person who was the spouse of a recipient of OAA, AB, or APTD, who was living with the recipient, and whose needs were included in the assistance payment, was eligible for Medicaid even though this "essential spouse" was not himself or herself eligible for public assistance.

The third and by far the most important optional group was the "medically needy." In this group were those individuals, otherwise eligible for money payments under the categorical assistance programs, whose income was above the standard of assistance (rendering them ineligible for assistance under these programs) but was inadequate to cover medical expenses. These were persons who would have qualified as "categorically needy" by virtue of being blind, elderly, disabled, or young except that their income fell above the cut-off level imposed in their state for cash assistance. Title XIX was unclear on how the "medically needy" were to be defined. States were required under the legislation to take into account the costs incurred for medical care when determining whether an individual was eligible for Medicaid. Exactly how this was to be done was not specified in the law, which merely noted that state standards should "provide for flexibility." Subsequent interpretation produced the "spend-down provision." In a state which chose to pick up the "medically needy" option, an individual became eligible for Medicaid payments as soon as he had spent on medical care the difference between his income and the state-determined eligibility level.

The legislation does not specifically state to which group(s) of recipients this provision refers. Analysis of the standards of eligibility suggests that only the medically needy were to be allowed to "spend down," an interpretation upheld by the courts in 1970. Therefore, a person in a state whose Medicaid plan was minimal, providing services only for the "categorically needy," would lose all his Medicaid entitlements by earning a few dollars above the categorical (cash) assistance level. On the other hand, a person in a state that also provided for the "medically needy" would never lose his eligibility so long as he spent down to the appropriate medical assistance level.

Eligibility for Nursing Home Care. Single adults in states having medically needy Medicaid programs with spend-down provisions were eligible for institutional care coverage if their income was less than the level at which their care was reimbursed under Medicaid. This was the case because all persons whose income was less than the level at which their care was reimbursed under Medicaid would obviously spend themselves down into eligibility. The reimbursement level rather than the regular Medicaid eligibility level thus became the effective eligibility level income for institutionalized persons under Medicaid in states with medically needy provisions. Persons with higher incomes could also spend down into eligibility, but since their income exceeded the cost of their care, they would not receive payments for it under Medicaid.

The situation was different in states without medically needy programs (and thus without spend-down provisions). In these states, all those people with incomes above the eligibility level but below the cost of institutional care were unable to purchase care through the Medicaid program. Many states created a special, higher standard of assistance for nursing home care so as to narrow this gap, however.

Under Medicaid regulations, patients were required to contribute financial assets in excess of a state-determined amount before Medicaid would contribute to care costs. Houses were treated differently. States normally provided for the retention of a community residence but in some instances this protection was waived for permanently institutionalized persons.

Eligibility for Medicaid coverage of at least part of the cost of nursing home care in a spend-down state for a married adult extended to an income (for the couple) equal to the cost of care plus an amount established by the state which was protected for the maintenance of the spouse remaining in the community. The couple was required to contribute an amount equal to the excess of care costs over the maintenance amounts allowed for the community and institutionalized persons. The treatment of couples in non-spend-down states paralleled the eligibility and payment treatment accorded single individuals in those states (that is, the standard of assistance for a two-person household was applied to the couple's combined income in determining either individual's eligibility).

Financial assets of couples were treated in the same fashion as those of individuals. Federal law, however, left no options to the states in the treatment of the homes of couples and required that they be protected—that is, that they not be claimed for payment of care.

Relative Responsibility. Financial responsibility of relatives was limited to a married recipient's spouse or a minor recipient's parent.[6] Title XIX prohibited states from subjecting other relatives to means tests as some states had done in determining MAA eligibility. Children could no longer be held responsible for elderly parents.

Reimbursement Policy. Title XIX as enacted in 1965 was vague on reimbursement policy. Nursing homes were to be reimbursed according to state policies which were to provide "such safeguards as may be necessary to assure that such care and services will be provided, in a manner consistent with simplicity of administration and the best interests of the recipients." States were advised by HEW that the fee structure should focus on a reasonable-cost basis, equivalent to the reimbursement methods under Part A of XVIII. Most states, however, departed from Title XVIII principles by imposing maximums on payments determined by reasonable cost, by paying uniform rates to all homes, and in other ways.

Federal regulations governing payment of Medicaid providers stipulated that "participation in the program will be limited to providers of service who accept, as payment in full, the amounts paid in accordance with the fee structure."[7] An exception was made, however, in the case of nursing homes in states with existing supplementation programs (states which allowed nursing homes to require medicaid recipients to supplement the state's reimbursement). These states were given until 1971 to provide HEW with a plan for phasing out supplementation within a "reasonable period." By 1974, providers in all states were required to accept Medicaid reimbursement as full payment. The providers in at least one state, however, devised a means of circumventing the law. In Florida, as the amount which the state would allow nursing homes to charge recipients diminished, some homes began to require families to make "contributions" (to the home's building or recreation fund, for example). A large majority of the state's homes have solicited and received such contributions, although apparently only a very few have violated a 1972 state law by making such contributions a condition of admission or proper care.

Federal/State Cost Sharing Arrangements. The federal government paid the "Federal Medical Assistance Percentage" of each state's Medicaid expenditures. Federal Medical Assistance was as follows:

$$100\% - \left[45\% \times \frac{(\text{state per capita income})^2}{(\text{national per capita income})^2} \right]$$

with a minimum of 50 percent set for states which by the formula would receive less, and a maximum of 83 percent set for states which by the formula would receive more.[8] Title XIX also provided that if the matching Federal Medical Assistance Percentage for any state, as computed by this formula, was less than 105 percent of the federal share of the medical expenditures made by the state during FY 1965, then 105 percent of the 1965 federal share should be the state's Federal Medical Assistance Percentage for FY 1966-1969.[9]

This was an improvement for the states over the MAA matching formula; not only did the formula for matching under Medicaid give a larger share to the federal government, with a maximum of 83 percent instead of the 80 percent allowed under MAA, but also, all states participating in Medicaid were guaranteed a federal share of 105 percent of the federal share of pre-Medicaid medical expenditures. The formula for federal share under MAA was as follows:

$$100\% - \left[50\% \times \frac{(\text{state per capita income})^2}{(\text{national per capita income})^2} \right]$$

Standards. The 1967 amendments to the Social Security Act prescribed general standards for Medicaid Skilled Nursing Homes and in so doing gave HEW the authority to write and enforce regulations implementing those standards. Prior to July 1970, when these regulations went into effect, SNHs were not required to comply with any legally enforceable federal standards. However, federal involvement in SNH standard-setting began earlier. The first standards for SNHs were published in June 1966, as supplement D to the Handbook of Public Assistance. These guidelines required that by January 1, 1968, SNHs meet the ECF staffing standards of (1) nursing service twenty-four hours a day, seven days a week; (2) an RN on the day shift, five days a week; and (3) a charge nurse on each shift with qualifications of one of two kinds—as an RN or as a Licensed Practical Nurse with a degree from a state-approved school of practical nursing. The guidelines served to tell the states how to interpret the provisions of Title XIX; they did not have the force of law. In March 1967, prior to the January 1968 compliance date, the staffing standards of Supplement D were revised to allow LPNs who were *not* graduates to qualify as charge nurses if (1) they had been acting successfully as charge nurses on July 1, 1967, and if (2) they had completed training satisfactory to the appropriate state licensing authority. The date of expected compliance was postponed a year to January 1, 1969.

In response to the standard-setting authority granted to it by the 1967 amendments to the Social Security Act, HEW issued Interim Policy Statement No. 19 in November 1968, two months before the implementation date specified in the legislation. The staffing requirements set forth in this statement were the same as those of the March 1967 version of Supplement D (RN full-time, at least a waivered LPN at all times). This policy statement served as advance notice of what was to be in the regulations implementing the SNH standards; its provisions did not carry the force of law. HEW failed to issue regulations by January 1969, when the SNH standards were to be implemented. Another Interim Policy Statement was issued in June 1969, in which the standards for charge nurses were made even less stringent (a nongraduate LPN was no longer required to have been acting as a charge nurse as of July 1, 1967, in order to qualify).

In April 1970, HEW issued final regulations for SNHs, the first federally enforceable SNH standards. These standards, effective July 1970, required Skilled Nursing Homes to be staffed at all times by a charge nurse with qualification of one of three kinds—as an RN or LPN with a degree from a state-approved school of practical nursing; as an LPN who, although not a graduate, had completed training satisfactory to the state licensing authority; or as an LPN who, although without a degree or equivalent training, had been successfully discharging the duties of a charge nurse on July 1, 1967. As required by the legislation, the 1967 Life Safety Code was also incorporated into these regulations. There was a significant variation across states, however, in the actual date of Life Safety Code enforcement. A number of states had incorporated the LSC or comparable requirements into their state nursing home licensure standards during the late 1950s or 1960s (though, typically, for new construction only); other states did not require full LSC compliance in new or existing facilities until the mid-1970s.

The standards for Medicaid skilled care facilities remained substantially unchanged until March 1974, when the regulations produced by the consolidation of Medicaid SNHs and Medicare ECFs went into effect. The new SNF standards required facilities to be staffed by an RN on the day shift seven days a week (rather than five) and by a charge nurse on all shifts with qualifications of one of two kinds—as a graduate RN or LPN or as a licensed LPN who, although not a graduate, possessed two years of appropriate experience following licensure and had passed a federally approved proficiency exam.

Intermediate Care. One of the 1967 Amendments to the Social Security Act, known as the Miller Amendment, authorized vendor payments to Intermediate Care Facilities under Title XI. States were given the option of adding ICF care to the benefits provided under each or any of their categorical assistance programs. Because long-term care at levels less intensive than skilled care could be made available to eligible recipients through OAA vendor payments in non-Medicaid

states, the addition of a Title XI ICF program to the OAA program did not
significantly affect the availability of ICF care for the elderly in these states. In
Medicaid states, however, the creation of the Title XI ICF program was
potentially significant. For the first time since its adoption of Medicaid, a state
participating in the Title XI ICF program could receive federal participation in
vendor payments for nursing home care less intensive than that provided in an
SNH. Prior to January 1968, when federal sharing of payments to ICFs under
Title XI began, Medicaid vendor payments to *skilled* nursing homes were the
only federal contribution to the cost of vendor payments for nursing home care
in Medicaid states. Most state OAA and MAA vendor payment programs covered
a range of nursing home care levels; thus a state's adoption of Medicaid
theoretically meant an abrupt end to payments to previously eligible facilities.
But in fact, most states allowed the majority of nursing homes to participate in
Title XIX, during the early years of Medicaid, at least, so that the adoption of an
ICF program usually resulted primarily in the downgrading of Medicaid SNHs
rather than in a significant increase in the number of facilities eligible for
participation in a federally funded vendor payment program.

In December 1971, ICFs were transferred to Title XIX, a move which
affected some aspects of the intermediate care program. A description of the
program as it functioned under both Titles follows.

Levels of Care Covered. Under Title XI, ICFs were to be defined and licensed by
the states; the category was to include institutions providing more than room
and board, but less than skilled nursing care. P.L. 92-223, the law transferring
ICFs from Title XI to Medicaid, defined an ICF as "an institution licensed under
State Law to provide, on a regular basis, health related care and services to
individuals who do not require the degree of care and treatment which a hospital
or skilled nursing home is designed to provide, but who because of their mental
or physical condition require care and services (above the level of room and
board) which can be made available to them only through institutional
services."[10]

Eligibility. Title XI stipulated that eligibility for ICF could be extended to
individuals who (1) were entitled (or would have been entitled if not in ICFs) to
receive money payments under one of the state categorical assistance programs;
(2) because of a physical or mental condition (or both), required living
accommodations and care which could be made available to them only through
institutional facilities; and (3) did not have such an illness, disease, injury, or
other condition as to require the degree of care and treatment which a hospital
or SNH was designed to provide.[11] In other words, ICF care was available to
those elderly persons meeting OAA financial eligibility criteria who needed
institutional care but not of the intensity provided in an SNH.

With the transfer of ICFs to Title XIX, states were given the option to extend eligibility for intermediate care to those persons whose incomes were too high to qualify them for cash assistance, but too low to cover medical costs—the medically needy. For a more detailed discussion of changes in the scope of eligibility resulting from the transfer of ICFs out of the categorical assistance programs into Medicaid, see the earlier section on eligibility for Medicaid skilled care. The changes in eligibility policy resulting from the shift of intermediate care into Medicaid paralleled the changes resulting from the shift of skilled care from OAA to Medicaid.

Reimbursement Policy. No reimbursement policy for ICF care was specified in Title XI. Title XIX authorized federal financial participation in payments to ICFs which on average did not exceed a ceiling of 90 percent of the statewide SNF rate. The HEW Regional Administrator of the Social and Rehabilitation Services Administration had the authority to grant exceptions to this rule. Typically, states reimbursed ICFs under both Titles XI and XIX according to SNF reimbursement policy, although ICF flat rates or ceilings were lower.

Federal/State Cost Sharing Arrangements. Title XI authorized federal sharing of vendor payments to ICFs in any state which modified its OAA plan (under Title I), AB plan (under Title X), APTD plan (under Title XIV), and/or AABD plan (under Title XII) to include ICF services. States received federal matching according to the formula used in federal matching under the categorical assistance programs except that states having a Medicaid program could elect to receive matching according to the Federal Medical Assistance Percentage used in federal matching under Title XIX. Because this arrangement brought a higher share from the federal government, most states with Medicaid programs elected to receive matching according to the Title XIX formula. With the transfer of ICFs to Title XIX, all states received matching according to the Federal Medical Assistance Percentage. The only exception was Arizona, which had no Medicaid program and therefore continued to provide ICF care under Title XI using the matching formula of the categorical assistance programs. The transfer to Title XIX affected federal/state cost-sharing arrangements for only the small number of states that although eligible to receive matching according to the Medicaid formula had opted for the categorical assistance formula instead.

Standards. Federal sharing of payments to ICFs began in January 1968; no federal standards for ICF care existed until HEW's Medical Services Administration issued Interim Policy Statement No. 23 in September 1968. The standards outlined in this statement did not carry the force of law; they served to give advance notice to the states of the content of the forthcoming regulations. In June 1969, the regulations were issued by HEW. A minimum range or level of care and services was mandated which included personal care and protective services, a responsible staff, assistance with "routine activities of daily living including such services as help in bathing, dressing, grooming, and management of personal affairs such as shopping." Social services, activities, health, preventive and physician services were to be provided by staff or through arrangement with outside agencies. Food services and special diets were to be provided, as well as reasonably private and decent living accommodations. The ICF was required to meet state laws governing licensure, and "such standards of safety and sanitation as are applicable to nursing homes under State Law."

These regulations established a system of what were essentially sheltered care accommodations for personal and social care, with assurances that health services should be available and provided as needed. A registered or licensed nurse was to be on duty during the day to deal with routine health problems.

State officials and others raised protests about these requirements and about the legality of the federal government's even issuing regulations without clearer legislative authorization. The result was that in June 1970 HEW published a greatly revised set of regulations which specified that the range or level of care and services now to be provided were to be left to the discretion of the states; the former requirements were reduced to recommended minimums.

When ICFs were transferred to Medicaid in 1971, the new section of Title XIX specified that "the term intermediate care facility means an institution which . . . meets such standards prescribed by the Secretary as he finds appropriate for the proper provision of such care. . . ." The federal government was thus given explicit standard-setting authority. ICFs, however, operated under Medicaid without federal standards until March 1974, when the regulations issued the previous month went into effect. The regulations specified requirements for the comfort and safety of the resident, covering such topics as fire safety (Life Safety Code), privacy, space, dining and recreation areas, linen, toilet facilities, and dietary services. Many of these requirements were not generally included in the state licensure standards which had previously governed ICFs. The new regulations contained more staffing requirements than the standards that had been in effect under Title XI. Supervision by a physician and a licensed pharmacist was required, at least on a consultant basis. Social services, activities programming, and dietary services were required. The standards required the facility to employ at least one full-time RN, or a full-time LPN with regular consultation (at least four hours weekly) from an RN. Waivered LPNs could qualify as charge nurses.

Although in some ways the new standards were more demanding than any that had been applied to ICFs in the past, the standards set forth in the regulations were generally vague and ambiguous. In requiring that ICF policies assure that "only those persons are accepted whose needs can be met by the facility directly or in cooperation with community resources or other providers of care with which it is affiliated or has contracts. . ." the regulations opened the door to widely varying levels of service provision among ICFs. Thus, the surveyor held and continues to hold discretionary power over what specific standards to apply to the individual facility.

Medicare

Title XVIII or Medicare, a federal health insurance program for the elderly, was added to the Social Security Act in October 1965. In January 1967, the federal government began making payments to nursing homes for extended care of Medicare beneficiaries.

Levels of Care Covered. Medicare paid for skilled care only. Medicare certified skilled care facilities were called Extended Care Facilities (ECFs). The definition of skilled care for the purposes of Medicare reimbursement was provided by the *Conditions of Participation* for Medicare ECFs.

Eligibility. In order to be eligible for Medicare, only had to be age sixty-five or over and eligible for retirement benefits under Title II (eligibility being earned through mandatory contributions to the Social Security trust fund) or under the railroad retirement system. Eligibility for nursing home care was limited to those who met the following requirements: prehospitalization for at least three days, admission within fourteen days of such hospital stay to a certified facility for the same condition which had required hospitalization, and physician's verification of the need for "skilled nursing" in continuation of care. A benefit limitation of 100 days was imposed, but most recipients became ineligible before reaching the maximum through failure to meet the need for skilled nursing requirement. Medicare covered the full cost of the first twenty days of ECF care; the recipient's coverage was subject to a coinsurance amount (equal to one-eighth of the inpatient hospital deductible) for each succeeding day.

In April 1969, the Bureau of Health Insurance (BHI) issued Intermediary Letter No. 370, which set forth new regulations on eligibility for Medicare extended care benefits. The above requirements were repeated but a new condition was added, requiring recipients to have "rehabilitation potential," effectively excluding coverage for terminal patients. These regulations also offered a revised and narrowed definition of the term "skilled nursing," which by statute was a precondition to coverage. Under the new definition, which spelled out with great specificity which medical and nursing services were covered, many patients were denied coverage, and these denials were given retroactive effect. In other words, a claim approved and paid prior to the issuance of the new definition could later be disallowed—with the nursing home or the patient required to make repayment.

The passage of the 1972 Amendments to the Social Security Act affected eligibility for extended care benefits in two ways. First, HEW was authorized to establish "presumptive periods of coverage" so that individuals with certain diagnoses upon discharge from the hospital would be "presumed" eligible for ECF care for a specific period. This provision put an end to the retroactive denials that had begun in 1969. Second, Medicare coverage was extended to those individuals under sixty-five who had been entitled to Social Security *disability* benefits for not less than twenty-four consecutive months.

Reimbursement Policy. "Principles of Reimbursement," a set of regulations issued by SSA, specified that ECFs were to be paid according to a "ratio of charges to charges applied to costs" formula, a reimbursement mechanism which placed no upper limit on nursing home costs. The method included a cost-plus factor for unidentifiable costs of 1.5 percent of gross costs for the proprietary nursing homes and 2 percent for nonprofit facilities. Interest costs, capital depreciation, and management expenses were all considered as allowable costs.

In 1969, at the same time that changes in Medicare eligibility policy resulted in retroactive denials, SSA began to implement direct cost control measures. The 1.5 percent cost-plus fee was removed, franchise fees were no longer considered as allowable costs, and the "prudent buyer" concept was adopted, limiting reimbursement to levels no higher than a prudent buyer would pay for similar services in a given geographic region. As well, the return on capital investment was limited to a return on the lowest of historical costs, fair market value, or current replacement minus straight line depreciation.

The passage of H.R. 1 (Public Law 92-603) in 1972 not only put an end to retroactive denials, but also eliminated another source of financial uncertainty for the provider. Prior to 1972, SSA had the authority to disallow incurred costs that were not reasonable. Because a number of problems inhibited the effective increase of this authority, providers were sometimes left without reimbursement for costs they had incurred. For example, the disallowance of costs after they had been incurred that were substantially out of line with those of comparable providers created financial uncertainty for the provider, since the provider had no way of knowing until sometime after he had incurred expenses whether or not they would be in line with expenses incurred by comparable providers in the same period. H.R. 1 helped put the provider on firmer ground by mandating that SSA's authority to disallow costs be exercised on a prospective rather than retrospective basis. Thus the provider would know in advance the limits to government recognition of incurred costs and would have the opportunity to act to avoid incurring nonreimbursable costs. The provider was further protected by the provision that (except with respect to emergency services) the beneficiary would be liable for the costs of items or services in excess of or more expensive than those determined to be necessary in the efficient delivery of needed health services.[12]

Standards. The first set of standards governing ECFs (entitled *Conditions of Participation for Medicare ECFs*) was issued by the Social Security Administration in May 1966. State health agencies were given responsibility for initial certification of ECFs and for the subsequent determination of compliance with the Conditions of Participation. The standards set forth in these regulations specified that ECFs provide (1) twenty-four-hour nursing service seven days a week, (2) a full-time RN (eight hours a day, five days a week) as director of nursing, (3) a charge nurse on each shift with qualifications of one of two kinds—as an RN or as a Licensed Practical Nurse with a degree from a state

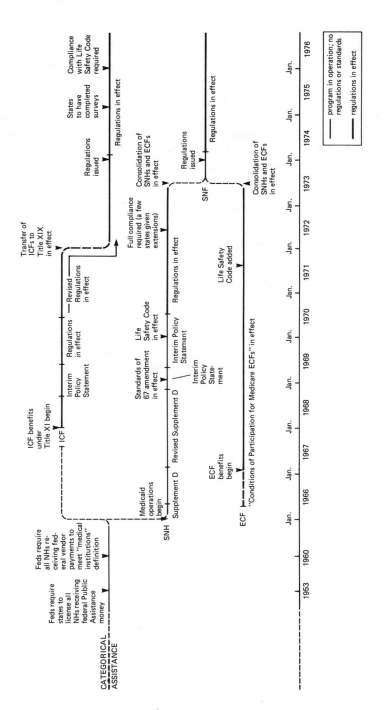

Figure B-1. Timeline of Federal Nursing Home Standards

approved school of practical nursing, and (4) sufficient other staff members to meet the requirements of the patients.

There were no major changes in the standards set forth in the Conditions of Participation until 1971 when the 1967 Life Safety Code was added. Then the standards remained substantially unchanged until March 1974, when the SNF regulations took effect requiring Medicare (and Medicaid) SNFs to be staffed by an RN eight hours a day, *seven* days a week rather than five, but permitting the use of a "waivered" LPN (a licensed LPN who, although not a graduate, had two years of appropriate experience following licensure and had passed a federally approved proficiency exam) as a charge nurse. The 1972 amendments to the Social Security Act, which included the provision for the consolidation of the standards for Medicare and Medicaid skilled nursing facilities, also authorized the granting of a special waiver of the RN requirement for SNFs in rural areas provided that the facility was without an RN for no more than two day shifts a week and that the facility made good-faith efforts to obtain another RN on a part-time basis.

Chronology: Legislative, Administrative, and Regulatory Federal Policy toward Nursing Homes and Related Facilities, 1950-1974

1950   Federal matching of medical vendor payments under OAA begun.

1953   As a condition for receiving federal matching funds for welfare purposes, each state required to designate standard-setting authorities to establish and maintain standards for medical institutions serving the recipient population.

1954   Hill-Burton Program amended to provide grants specifically for the construction of public and voluntary nonprofit nursing homes.

1956   Social Security Act amended so that federal matching funds available for medical assistance are no longer limited by the monthly dollar ceiling amounts per individual recipient applicable in the matching formula for cash assistance payments. Loan program for proprietary nursing homes inauguarated by Small Business Administration.

1959   Mortgage insurance program for proprietary nursing homes established by Congress under the Federal Housing Authority.

1960   Kerr-Mills bill enacted providing increased federal matching for OAA vendor payments and creating MAA. All institutions receiving federal vendor payments required to meet "medical institutions" definition.

1961   OAA per-recipient vendor payment addition subject to federal matching increased from $12 to $15.

1965   Some MAA program in operation in forty-four of fifty-four jurisdictions. Titles XVIII and XIX added to the Social Security Act.

1966

Jan.   Medicaid operations begun (onset of vendor payments to nursing homes may have occurred somewhat later).

May   Conditions of Participation for Medicare ECFs issued by the Social Security Administration. (Standards in effect until 3/8/74.)

June   Guidelines for Medicaid SNHs published as Supplement D to the Handbook of Public Assistance.

1967

Jan.   Extended care benefits under Medicare begun; 2,800 facilities certified as in full or substantial compliance.

Mar.   Staffing standards of Supplement D revised; LPNs who are *not* graduates can qualify as charge nurses under certain conditions.

July   All operating Medicaid programs required to provide vendor payments for SNH care (prior to July 1, participating states were required only to provide "some institutional service.")

Oct.   "Principles of Reimbursement" of ECF Conditions of Participation amended to include a "return on investment factor."

Dec.   Amendments to the Social Security Act:

          1. Vendor payments to ICFs under Title XI authorized (effective 1/1/68).
          2. Medical review of Medicaid skilled nursing home care required (effective 7/1/69).
          3. SNHs required to meet Life Safety Code (effective 1/1/70).
          4. States directed to make periodic on-site inspections of SNHs.
          5. SNH standards prescribed (effective 1/1/69, no regulations implementing standards issued until 4/1/70).
          6. Licensure of administrators of SNHs required (effective 7/1/70).

1968

Jan.   Federal sharing of payments to ICFs begun.

Sept.   Interim Policy Statement containing standards for ICFs issued by MSA.

Nov.   Interim Policy Statement on SNH standards, repeating the standards of
        the March 1967 version of Supplement D, issued by HEW.

1969

Jan.   1967 amendment prescribing SNH standards effective requiring:

        1. disclosure of ownership;
        2. organization and supervision of nursing services;
        3. meal and dietary planning services;
        4. provision for medical supervision, medical records, drug adminis-
            tration, emergency care; and
        5. arrangements with hospitals for diagnosis and acute care hospital
            services.

Apr.   Intermediary Letter detailing Covered Care Guidelines issued by BHI:
        retroactive denials of Medicare ECF care begun.

June   Interim Policy Statement on SNH standards issued by MSA; charge
        nurse standards made less stringent (effective 7/1/70). Regulations on
        ICF standards issued by MSA.

July   Medical review requirement for SNH care effective.

Dec.   1967 amendment requiring SNHs to meet standards designed to protect
        the health and safety of patients effective.

1970

Jan.   1967 amendment requiring SNHs to meet Life Safety Code effective.
        Federal sharing of vendor payments under OAA, AFDC, AB, APTD,
        AABD, and MAA ended.

Apr.   Final regulations for SNHs issued by MSA (effective 7/1/70).

June   ICF regulations revised; states to determine standards on range or level
        of care and services.

July   MSA regulations on SNH standards effective (standards remain substan-
        tially unchanged until 3/8/74). States required to establish programs for
        the licensing of nursing home administrators.

1971

Aug.   Statement issued by President Nixon in New Hampshire calling for
        major federal effort in reviewing LTC.

Oct.   ECF Conditions of Participation amended to include Life Safety Code.

Nov.   Announcement made by HEW Secretary Elliot Richardson that there
        will be no federal support of substandard homes; states required to
        complete certification of all Medicaid SNHs (effective 7/1/72).

Dec.   Social Security Act amended transferring ICFs to Title XIX.

1972

Jan.   Reimbursements to ICFs under Title XIX begun ("medically needy"
        become eligible for ICF care).

July   Special unit to deal with nursing homes established in each HEW
        regional office. Cut-off of federal support to substandard SNHs effec-
        tive.

Oct.   Amendments to Social Security Act:

        1. A single definition and set of standards for ECFs under Medicare
           and SNHs under Medicaid established, the resulting "skilled nursing
           facilities" (SNFs) eligible to participate in Medicare and Medicaid
           (effective 7/1/73, no regulations implementing provision issued
           until 1/1/74).
        2. Definitions of care requirements for extended care benefits under
           Medicare and skilled nursing care under Medicaid made the same
           (effective 1/1/73).
        3. RN nursing requirement for SNFs in rural areas waived under
           certain conditions.
        4. 100 percent federal reimbursement for costs of survey and inspec-
           tion of SNFs and ICFs under Medicaid extended through 6/30/74.
        5. Federal participation in reimbursement for Medicaid skilled and
           intermediate care per diem costs limited to 105 percent of prior
           year's level of payments (effective 1/1/73).
        6. States required to reimburse SNFs and ICFs on a "reasonable
           cost-related" basis (effective 7/1/76).
        7. "Presumed Coverage" provisions end Medicare retroactive denials.
        8. Medicare eligibility extended to individuals over sixty-five eligible
           for Social Security disability benefits.
        9. PSROs created.

1973

Jan.   Limits on payments to Medicaid facilities effective. Consolidation of
        definitions of skilled care under Medicare and Medicaid effective.

July   Consolidation of ECFs and SNHs into a single category (SNFs)
        effective.

1974

Jan.   Regulations on standards for SNFs and ICFs issued by HEW (effective 3/8/74).

Mar.   SNF and ICF regulations effective.

Notes

1. Social Security Act, Title I, Section 2, (b).
2. P.L. 86-788, Section 601 (c).
3. P.L. 83-788, Section 601 (a).
4. P.L. 83-788, Sections 601 (a) and (b).
5. P.L. 86-788, Section 601 (c).
6. Social Security Act, Title XIX, Section 2 (a).
7. 45 Code of Federal Regulations, 250.30 (a) (8).
8. Social Security Act, Title XIX, Section 3 (a).
9. Social Security Act, Title XIX, Section 3 (c).
10. Social Security Act, Title XIX, Section 5 (c).
11. Social Security Act, Title XI, Section 21 (b).
12. P.L. 92-603, Section 203.

Bibliography

Markus, Glenn R. *Nursing Homes and the Congress: A Brief History of Developments and Issues.* Washington, D.C.: Congressional Research Service, 1972.

Russell, Louise B., et al. *Federal Health Spending: 1969-1974.* Washington, D.C.: Center for Health Policy Studies, National Planning Association, 1974.

Old Age Assistance and Medical Assistance for the Aged

Congressional Quarterly Service. "History of Medical Care Proposals, 1945-1964." *Congress and the Nation, 1945-1964,* Volume I. Washington, D.C.: Congressional Quarterly Service, 1965.

Moroney, Robert M., and Kurtz, Norman R. "The Evolution of Long-Term Care Institutions." In Sylvia Sherwood, ed. *Long-Term Care: A Handbook for Researchers, Planners and Providers.* New York: Spectrum Publications, 1975.

Stevens, Robert, and Stevens, Rosemary. *Welfare Medicine in America: A Case Study of Medicaid.* New York: The Free Press, 1974.

U.S. Congress. Senate. Special Committee on Aging. *Eighteen Months of Experience with the Medical Assistance for the Aged (Kerr-Mills) Program.* 87th Cong., 2nd sess., 1962.

U.S. Congress. Senate. Special Committee on Aging. Subcommittee on Health of the Elderly. *Medical Assistance for the Aged, the Kerr-Mills Program, 1960-1963.* 88th Cong., 1st sess., 1963.

U.S. Department of Health, Education and Welfare. Social and Rehabilitative Services. *Characteristics of State Medical Assistance Programs Under Title XIX of the Social Security Act.* Public Assistance Series No. 49, 1970.

U.S. Department of Health, Education and Welfare. Social and Rehabilitative Services. *Characteristics of State Public Assistance Plans Under the Social Security Act: Provisions for Medical and Remedial Care.* Public Assistance Report No. 49, 1962, 1964.

U.S. Department of Health, Education and Welfare. Social and Rehabilitative Services. *1964-1965 Supplement to Provisions for Medical and Remedial Care, Part II: Medical Assistance for the Aged.* Public Assistance Report No. 49-A, 1965.

Medicaid

Davison, Richard. "The Place of the Intermediate Care Facility in the Long-Term Care Spectrum." Mimeographed. Washington, D.C., 1972.

Frantz, Frank. "Characteristics of Titles XVIII and XIX Underlying Differences in Standards and Requirements." Paper presented at Bi-Regional Cooperative Conference of State and Federal Agencies, St. Petersburg, Florida, June 21, 1972.

Lavor, Judy. "Intermediate Care Facilities." Mimeographed. Washington, D.C.: U.S. Department of Health, Education and Welfare, 1974.

Markus, Glenn R. *Nursing Homes and the Congress: A Brief History of Developments and Issues.* Washington, D.C.: Congressional Research Service, 1972.

Pollak, William. "Expanding Eligibility on a Fee Basis Higher Up the Income Scale as a Part of Short-Term Medicaid Modification Strategy." Typewritten. Washington, D.C., 1974.

Stevens, Robert, and Stevens, Rosemary. *Welfare Medicine in America: A Case Study of Medicaid.* New York: The Free Press, 1974.

U.S. Department of Health, Education and Welfare. Social and Rehabilitative Services. *Characteristics of State Medical Assistance Programs Under Title XIX of the Social Security Act.* Public Assistance Series No. 49, 1970.

Medicare

Markus, Glenn R. *Nursing Homes and the Congress: A Brief History of Developments and Issues.* Washington, D.C.: Congressional Research Service, 1972.

Spitz, Bruce. "Nursing Homes and Prospective Reimbursement." Working Paper 5057-2. Washington, D.C.: The Urban Institute, 1976.

Stevens, Robert, and Stevens, Rosemary. *Welfare Medicine in America: A Case Study of Medicaid.* New York: The Free Press, 1974.

U.S. Department of Health, Education and Welfare. Social Security Administration. *Your Medicare Handbook,* 1975.

Appendix C:
Comparison of NCHS and State Nursing Home Data

The National Center for Health Statistics classifies nursing homes and related facilities into four categories: Nursing Care Homes, Personal Care Homes with Nursing, Personal Care Homes without Nursing, and Domiciliary Care Homes. These facilities are defined on the basis of the primary or predominant service offered as follows:

1. A nursing care home is defined as one in which 50 percent or more of the residents receive one or more nursing services and the facility has at least one registered nurse (RN) or licensed practical nurse (LPN) employed thirty-five or more hours per week. Nursing services include nasal feeding, catheterization, irrigation, oxygen therapy, full bed bath, enema, hypodermic injection, intravenous injection, temperature-pulse-respiration, blood pressure, application of dressing or bandage, or bowel and bladder retraining.
2. A personal care home with nursing care is defined as one in which either (a) some, but less than 50 percent, of the residents receive nursing care or, (b) more than 50 percent of the residents receive nursing care, but no RNs or LPNs are employed full time on the staff.
3. A personal care home is defined as one in which the facility routinely provides three or more of the following personal services but no nursing service. Personal services include rub or massage service or assistance with bathing, dressing, correspondence or shopping, walking or getting about, or eating.
4. A domiciliary care home is defined as one in which the facility routinely provides less than three of the personal services specified in the definition above, and no nursing service. This type of facility provides a sheltered environment primarily for persons who are able to care for themselves.

In our collection and treatment of nursing home data in the ten sample states, we chose to include whatever the state licensure agency defined as a nursing home. Operationally this almost always corresponded to those licensure categories out of which the state certified facilities for participation in the Medicaid program as SNFs or ICFs.

A comparison of NCHS and Urban Institute data for individual states reveals that for both beds and facilities, data reflecting the aggregate of the NCHS "nursing care" and "personal care with nursing" categories more closely approximate overall the data collected in the states than do data on the NCHS "nursing care" category alone in 1967 and 1969. While in serveral states, the figure for the top NCHS category alone was a better approximation of the figure obtained in the state than the figure resulting from the addition of the top two NCHS categories, on average, the aggregate figure was more accurate (see table C-1).

For 1971 and 1973, however, NCHS data for the "nursing care" category alone more closely resemble UI-collected data than do data reflecting the aggregate of the top two NCHS categories. One might expect to find that in 1971 state figures and previously comparable NCHS figures began to diverge, because between 1969 and 1971 many states instituted more demanding licensure standards, or, with the help of Medicaid money which became available to state survey agencies at that time, began to enforce previously unenforced standards. Consequently, while the criteria used in defining the NCHS nursing home categories remained unchanged, many facilities increased their staffing levels and thus shifted up into a higher NCHS category. As can be seen in the table, this upward shift of facilities was enough to bring the figures on the single NCHS "nursing care" category into line with state licensure figures.

Based on a comparison of NCHS and UI-collected state data, then, it appears that in comparisons of national and individual state nursing home utilization levels, national data should be derived by combining the NCHS "nursing care" and "personal care with nursing" categories for 1967 and 1969, and by using the "nursing care" category alone for 1971 and 1973.

Table C-1
Comparison of NCHS and State Licensure Figures for Nursing Home Beds and Facilities

	Beds				Facilities			
	1967	1969	1971	1973[c]	1967	1969	1971	1973[c]
Alabama								
% NCHS NC # is of state #	82	89	98	93	74	88	98	92
% NCHS NC + PC w/N # is of state #	91	93	104	NA[d]	85	93	104	NA
California								
NC	90	100	112	120	87	99	116	136
NC + PC w/N	117	119	131	NA	127	134	155	NA
Florida								
NC	91	83	112	100	88	90	105	100
NC + PC w/N	117	96	128	NA	104	100	120	NA
Mississippi								
NC	83	69	85	94	90	75	87	93
NC + PC w/N	104	80	93	NA	122	94	100	NA
New Jersey								
NC	81	89	102	111	78	84	90	108
NC + PC w/N	104	110	117	NA	101	106	110	NA
New York								
NC	93	78	91	83	95	76	84	91
NC + PC w/N	120	103	114	NA	128	104	109	NA
South Dakota								
NC	75	71	78	98	73	74	75	94
NC + PC w/N	114	97	106	NA	120	102	109	NA
Vermont								
NC	92	95	104	112	90	89	95	125
NC + PC w/N	111	111	118	NA	112	113	124	NA

West Virginia								
NC	89[a]	97[a]	116	137	NA[b]	NA[b]	119	144
NC + PC w/N	120[a]	129[a]	146	NA	NA[b]	NA[b]	167	NA
Wisconsin								
NC	71	77	93	94	58	68	82	95
NC + PC w/N	94	94	115	NA	86	91	106	NA
Ten-state mean								
NC	85	85	99	104	82	83	95	108
NC + PC w/N	109	103	117	>104	109	104	120	>108

[a]Since no data were available in West Virginia on the number of nursing home beds in these years, estimates were made using the average annual increase in number of beds between 1964 and 1970.

[b]No data were available in West Virginia on the number of nursing homes in these years, and no estimates could be made because the pattern of growth during the years for which data were available was so irregular.

[c]No data are available on numbers of beds or facilities in the "personal care home with nursing" category for 1973.

[d]NA = Not Available.

**Appendix D:
Sample State Nursing
Home and Supportive
Residential Facility
Bed Data**

Table D-1
Bed Supply: Alabama

	1961	1962	1963	1964	1965	1966	1967	1968	1969	1970	1971	1972	1973	1974
Skilled Nursing Homes/SNFs														
Number	1,565	2,253	3,350	4,715	6,568	7,908	8,561	9,862	11,435	10,881	9,182	7,859	10,613	11,683
% of Total	46.2	55.2	66.7	75.3	84.3	87.4	88.8	93.4	95.4	86.9	71.8	57.5	69.9	69.9
% Increase	—	44.0	48.7	40.7	39.3	20.4	8.3	15.2	16.0	-4.8	-15.6	-14.4	35.0	10.1
Nursing Homes/ICFs														
Number	1,826	1,830	1,676	1,543	1,225	1,137	1,085	695	548	1,646	3,602	5,809	4,578	5,020
% of Total	53.8	44.8	33.3	24.7	15.7	12.6	11.2	6.6	4.6	13.1	28.2	42.5	30.1	30.1
% Increase	—	0.2	-8.4	-7.9	-20.6	-7.2	-4.6	-35.9	-21.2	200.4	118.8	61.3	-21.2	9.7
Total														
Number	3,391	4,083	5,026	6,258	7,793	9,045	9,646	10,557	11,983	12,527	12,784	13,668	15,191	16,703
% Increase Beds	—	20.4	23.1	24.5	24.5	16.1	6.6	9.4	13.5	4.5	2.1	6.9	11.1	10.0
Beds per 100 Aged	1.27	1.50	1.83	2.24	2.70	3.07	3.19	3.42	3.83	3.87	3.78	3.93	4.28	4.58
% Inc. Beds/100 Aged	—	18.1	22.0	22.4	20.5	13.7	3.9	7.2	12.0	1.0	-2.3	4.0	8.9	7.0
65+ Pop. (in 100s)	268	272	275	279	289	295	302	309	313	324	338	348	355	365
% Increase 65+ Pop.	—	1.5	1.1	1.5	3.6	2.1	2.4	2.3	1.3	3.5	4.3	3.0	2.0	2.8
Personal Care Homes														
Number	NA[a]	NA	310	322	291	268	247	321	433	398	439	433	485	485
% Increase	—	—	—	3.9	-9.6	-7.9	-7.8	30.0	34.9	-8.1	10.3	-1.4	12.0	0.0
Beds per 100 Aged	—	—	0.1	0.1	0.1	0.0	0.0	0.1	0.1	0.1	0.1	0.1	0.1	0.1
Proprietary Nursing Home Beds														
Number	NA	NA	NA	NA	NA	7,158	7,525	8,327	9,705	10,130	10,367	11,161	12,518	13,955
% of Total	—	—	—	—	—	79.1	78.0	78.9	81.0	81.1	81.7	81.7	82.4	83.5
% Increase	—	—	—	—	—	—	5.1	10.7	16.6	4.4	2.3	7.7	12.2	11.5

Nonprofit
Nursing
Home Beds

Number	NA	NA	NA	NA	1,887	2,121	2,230	2,278	2,397	2,417	2,507	2,673	2,748
% of Total	—	—	—	—	20.9	22.0	21.1	19.0	18.9	18.3	18.3	17.6	16.5
% Increase	—	—	—	—	—	12.4	5.1	2.1	5.2	0.8	3.7	6.6	2.8

[a]NA = Not Available.

Table D-2
Bed Supply: California

	1960	1961	1962	1963	1964	1965
Nursing Home Beds						
Number[a]	16,819	18,735	22,264	27,829	36,351	43,573
% Increase—Beds	–	11.4	11.9	25.0	30.6	19.9
Beds per 100 Aged	1.22	1.31	1.52	1.81	2.36	2.76
% Increase—Beds/100 Aged	–	7.4	16.0	19.1	30.4	17.0
65+ Pop. (in 1,000s)	1,376	1,429	1,469	1,505	1,541	1,576
% Increase—65+ Pop.	–	3.9	2.8	2.6	2.4	2.3
Personal Care Home Beds						
Boarding Number	NA[f]	NA	NA	NA	NA	NA
Homes % Increase	–	–	–	–	–	–
for the Beds/100 Aged	–	–	–	–	–	–
Aged[c]						
Institu- Number	NA	NA	NA	NA	NA	NA
tions % Increase	–	–	–	–	–	–
for the Beds/100 Aged	–	–	–	–	–	–
Aged[d]						
Long-Term Care Private Mental						
Health Facility Beds[e]						
Number	NA	NA	NA	NA	NA	NA
% Increase	–	–	–	–	–	–
Beds/100 Aged	–	–	–	–	–	–

[a]Bed counts reflect censuses as of March in years 1960-1965 and in 1969; June in 1966 and 1968; July in 1970; December in 1972 and 1973; September in 1974.

[b]Approximate.

[c]Facilities of fewer than 16 beds and licensed by the County Boards of Social Welfare. No nursing care is provided.

1966	1967	1968	1969	1970	1971	1972	1973	1974
53,988	58,949[b]	68,200	75,631	92,166[b]	95,220[b]	96,765	96,601	97,777
23.9	9.2	15.7	10.9	21.9	3.3	1.6	−0.2	1.2
3.36	3.58	4.03	4.40	5.14	5.14	5.12	4.99	4.92
21.7	6.6	12.6	9.2	16.8	0	−0.4	−2.5	−1.4
1,606	1,645	1,692	1,719	1,792	1,851	1,888	1,935	1,986
1.9	2.4	2.9	1.6	4.3	3.3	2.0	2.5	2.6
NA	NA	NA	NA	NA	NA	21,154	21,685	22,462
−	−	−	−	−	−	−	2.5	3.6
−	−	−	−	−	−	1.12	1.12	1.13
NA	NA	NA	26,548	29,507	NA	NA	NA	NA
−	−	−	−	11.2	−	−	−	−
−	−	−	1.54	1.65	−	−	−	−
NA	NA	6,757	NA	NA	9,339	9,964	9,643	9,342
−	−	−	−	−	−	6.7	−3.2	−3.1
−	−	0.40	−	−	0.50	0.53	0.50	0.47

[d]Facilities of 16 or more beds or institutional in character and licensed by the State Department of Social Welfare until 1973 and by the Health Department since 1973. No nursing care is provided.

[e]These facilities resemble nursing homes in many respects but provide specialized services for the mentally ill and are permitted locks on room and ward doors.

[f]NA = Not Available.

Table D-3
Bed Supply: Florida

	1962	1963	1964	1965	1966	1967	1968	1969	1970	1971	1972	1973	1974
Nursing Home Beds													
Number	9,553	10,975	13,468	14,983	16,657	18,339	21,557	23,062	25,400	26,607	27,956	29,262	29,796
% Increase—Beds	–	14.9	22.7	11.3	11.2	10.1	17.6	7.0	10.1	4.8	5.1	4.7	1.8
Beds per 100 Aged	1.53	1.68	1.96	2.13	2.25	2.39	2.61	2.73	2.58	2.50	2.48	2.45	2.35
% Increase—Beds/100 Aged	–	9.8	16.7	8.7	5.6	6.2	9.2	4.6	–5.5	–3.1	–0.8	–1.2	–4.1
65+ Pop. (1,000s)	626	655	686	703	739	767	824	846	985	1,065	1,127	1,196	1,267
% Increase—65+ Pop.	–	4.6	4.7	2.5	5.1	3.8	7.4	2.7	16.4	8.1	5.8	6.1	5.9
Home for the Aged Beds													
Number	1,404	1,345	2,480	2,192	4,155	4,334	5,582	9,103	8,775	10,063	13,923	15,740	3,964[a]
% Increase	–	–4.2	84.4	–11.6	89.6	4.3	28.8	63.1	–3.6	14.7	38.4	13.1	–74.8
Beds per 100 Aged	0.22	0.21	0.36	0.32	0.56	0.57	0.68	1.08	0.89	0.94	1.24	1.32	0.31
Proprietary Nursing Home Beds[b]													
Number	NA	NA	NA	NA	NA	NA	18,178	19,212	21,082	21,704	22,719	23,416	23,727
% of Total	–	–	–	–	–	–	84.3	83.3	83.0	81.6	81.3	80.0	79.6
% Increase	–	–	–	–	–	–	–	5.7	9.7	2.9	4.7	3.1	1.3
Nonprofit Voluntary Nursing Home Beds[b]													
Number	NA	NA	NA	NA	NA	NA	2,582	2,929	3,444	4,044	4,433	4,845	4,902
% of Total	–	–	–	–	–	–	12.0	12.7	13.6	15.2	15.9	16.6	16.5
% Increase	–	–	–	–	–	–	–	1.3	17.6	17.4	9.6	9.3	1.2
Public Nursing Home Beds[b]													
Number	NA	NA	NA	NA	NA	NA	797	921	874	859	804	1,001	1,167
% of Total	–	–	–	–	–	–	3.7	4.0	3.4	3.2	2.9	3.4	3.9
% Increase	–	–	–	–	–	–	–	15.6	–5.1	–1.7	–6.4	24.5	16.6

[a]The significant decrease in number of beds from the previous year resulted from the transfer of the bulk of the Homes for the Aged into a newly created category, Residential Homes for the Aged, under the authority of the Division of Hotels and Restaurants.
[b]Figures reflect the number of nursing home beds of each ownership type; Home for the Aged beds are not included.
[c]NA = Not Available.

Table D-4
Bed Supply: Mississippi[a]

	1963	1964	1965	1966	1967	1968	1969	1970	1971	1972	1973	1974
Intensive and Skilled Care												
Number	2,797	2,811	2,853	1,097	1,927	2,652	3,500	4,786	5,036	5,406	5,858	6,757
% of Total				37.2	58.4	65.3	70.5	71.8	66.5	69.6	73.4	76.0
% Increase	—			—	75.7	37.6	32.0	36.7	5.2	7.4	8.4	15.4
		includes beds in intensive, skilled, intermediate, and personal care homes										
Intermediate Care												
Number				1,741	1,224	1,118	1,128	1,213	1,725	1,716	1,408	1,417
% of Total				59.1	37.1	27.5	22.7	13.2	22.8	22.1	17.6	15.9
% Increase		—		—	-29.7	-8.7	0.9	7.5	42.2	-0.5	-18.1	0.6
Extended Care												
Number	110	110	110	110	150	290	340	670	810	650	717	718
% of Total	4.2	4.2	4.2	3.7	4.5	7.1	6.8	10.0	10.7	8.4	9.0	8.1
% Increase	—	0	0	0	36.4	9.3	17.2	9.7	20.9	-19.7	10.3	0.1
Total												
Number	2,600[b]	2,625[b]	2,650[b]	2,948	3,301	4,060	4,968	6,669	7,571	7,772	7,983	8,892
% Increase—Beds	—	1.0	1.0	11.2	12.0	23.0	22.4	34.2	13.5	2.7	2.7	11.4
Beds per 100 Aged	1.32	1.33	1.30	1.43	1.56	1.90	2.29	3.02	3.29	3.31	3.33	3.61
% Increase—Beds/100 Aged	—	0.8	-2.3	9.2	10.0	21.8	20.5	31.9	8.9	0.6	0.6	8.4
65+ Pop. (in 1,000s)	197	198	204	207	211	214	217	221	230	235	240	246
% Increase—65+ Pop.	—	0.5	3.0	1.5	1.9	1.4	1.4	1.8	4.1	2.2	2.1	2.5
Personal Care												
Number	NA[d]	NA	NA	324	275	213	211	171	274	274	275	260
% Increase	—	—	—	—	-15.1	-22.6	-0.01	-19.0	60.2	0	0.4	-5.4
Beds per 1,000 Aged	—	—	—	0.16	0.13	0.10	0.10	0.08	0.12	0.12	0.15	0.11
Proprietary[c]												
Nursing Home Beds												
Number	NA	NA	NA	NA	2,214	2,640	3,447	4,711	5,188	5,526	5,643	6,252
% of Total	—	—	—	—	67.1	65.0	69.4	70.6	68.5	71.1	70.7	70.3
% Increase	—	—	—	—	—	19.2	30.6	36.7	10.3	6.5	2.1	10.8

Table D-4 continued

	1963	1964	1965	1966	1967	1968	1969	1970	1971	1972	1973	1974
Nonprofit Voluntary Nursing Home Beds[c]												
Number	NA	NA	NA	NA	650	751	852	790	762	745	689	741
% of Total	–	–	–	–	19.7	18.5	17.2	11.9	10.1	7.6	8.6	8.3
% Increase	–	–	–	–	–	15.5	13.4	-7.3	-3.5	-2.2	-7.5	7.6
Public Nursing Home Beds[c]												
Number	NA	NA	NA	NA	437	669	669	1,168	1,621	1,501	1,651	1,899
% of Total	–	–	–	–	13.2	16.5	13.5	17.5	21.4	19.3	20.7	21.4
% Increase	–	–	–	–	–	53.1	0	74.6	38.8	7.4	10.0	15.0

[a]Figures reflect the number of licensed beds on December 31 of each year 1963-1966; July 31 of each year 1967-1974.

[b]Figures are estimates derived by subtracting 300 (a rough approximation of the number of personal care beds) from the total.

[c]Figures reflect the number of nursing home beds of each ownership type; personal care beds are not included.

[d]NA = Not Available.

Table D-5
Bed Supply: New Jersey

	1964	1965	1966	1967	1968	1969	1970	1971	1972	1973	1974
Beds in Nursing Homes	7,852	9,417	10,664	12,221	12,937	13,881	14,788	16,081	16,585	18,359	18,693
Beds in ICFs[b]	—	—	—	—	—	—	—	—	—	1,000	1,000
Nursing Home Beds in Homes for the Aged[b]	2,500	2,530	2,560	2,590	2,620	2,650	2,680	2,710	2,740	2,770	2,800
Nursing Home Beds in Hospitals[b]	450	425	400	375	350	325	300	275	250	225	195
Nursing Home Beds in Gov. Medical Institutions	3,000	3,000	3,000	3,000	3,000	3,000	3,000	3,000	3,000	3,000	3,000
Total Number of Beds[b]	13,802	15,372	16,624	18,186	18,907	19,856	20,768	22,066	22,375	25,354	25,688
% Increase Beds	—	11.4	8.1	9.4	4.0	5.0	6.0	6.3	1.4	13.3	1.3
Beds per 100 Aged	2.16	2.38	2.59	2.78	2.85	2.95	2.99	3.10	3.10	3.51	3.42
% Increase Beds/100 Aged	—	10.2	8.8	7.3	2.5	3.5	1.4	3.7	0	13.2	−2.6
65+ Pop. (in 1,000s)	617	629	641	653	664	674	694	711	722	734	749
% Increase 65+ Pop.	—	1.9	1.9	1.9	1.7	1.5	3.0	2.5	1.6	1.7	2.0
Beds in Boarding Homes for Sheltered Care[b]	NA[a]	500	1,677	2,854	4,037	5,208	6,385	7,562	8,740	9,916	11,000

[a]NA = Not Available.
[b]Estimates.

Table D-6
Bed Supply: New York[a]

	1964	1965	1966	1967	1968	1969	1970	1971	1972	1973	1974
Nursing Home/SNF											
Number	40,000	42,000	44,566	44,756	47,151	49,781	51,433	54,616	59,633	66,223	68,194
% of Total	100.0	100.0	100.0	100.0	100.0	80.8	80.7	81.5	81.2	80.8	77.5
% Increase	–	5.0	6.1	0.4	5.4	5.6	3.3	6.2	9.2	11.1	3.0
HRF/ICF											
Number		–	–	–	–	11,812	12,314	12,382	13,821	15,784	19,823
% of Total		–	–	–	–	19.2	19.3	18.5	18.8	19.2	22.5
% Increase		–	–	–	–	–	4.3	0.6	11.6	14.2	25.6
Total											
Number	40,000	42,000	44,566	44,756	47,151	61,593[d]	63,747	66,998	73,454	82,007	88,017
% Increase—Beds	–	5.0	6.1	0.4	5.4	30.6	3.5	5.1	9.6	11.6	7.3
Beds per 100 Aged	2.19	2.27	2.38	2.35	2.46	3.15	3.27	3.39	3.71	4.13	4.41
% Increase—Beds/100 Aged	–	3.7	4.9	–1.3	4.7	28.1	3.8	3.7	9.4	11.3	6.8
65+ Pop. (in 1,000s)	1,825	1,851	1,872	1,903	1,914	1,958	1,951	1,974	1,982	1,985	1,998
% Increase—65+ Pop.	–	1.4	1.1	1.7	0.6	2.3	–0.7	1.2	0.4	0.2	0.7
PPHA[b]											
Number	NA[e]	NA	NA	NA	NA	NA	NA	10,240	12,107	16,281	20,846
% Increase	–	–	–	–	–	–	–	–	18.2	34.5	28.0
Beds per 100 Aged	–	–	–	–	–	–	–	0.52	0.61	0.82	1.04
Proprietary Nursing Home Beds[c]											
Number	22,500	24,000	25,737	25,824	28,933	29,862	31,598	34,101	37,237	40,743	47,524
% of Total	56.3	57.1	57.8	57.7	61.4	48.5	49.6	50.9	50.7	49.7	54.0
% Increase	–	6.7	7.2	0.3	12.0	3.2	5.8	7.9	9.2	9.4	16.6
Nonprofit Voluntary Nursing Home Beds[c]											
Number	NA	–	9,354	9,607	8,853	18,106	18,726	19,806	22,233	27,320	26,532
% of Total	–	–	21.0	21.5	18.8	29.4	29.4	29.6	30.3	33.3	30.1
% Increase	–	–	–	2.7	–7.9	104.5	3.4	5.8	12.3	22.9	2.9

Public Nursing Home Beds[c]

Number	NA	NA	9,475	9,325	9,365	13,625	13,423	13,091	13,984	13,944	13,961
% of Total	—	—	21.3	20.8	19.9	22.1	21.1	19.5	19.0	17.0	15.9
% Increase	—	—	—	-1.6	0.4	45.5	-1.5	-2.5	6.8	0.3	0.1

[a]Figures reflect census as of October or September of each year except 1970, for which figures reflect the June census.

[b]The only category of Domiciliary Care Facilities for which data were available was Private Proprietary Homes for Adults; however, the vast majority of DCFs are classified as PPHAs.

[c]Figures reflect the number of nursing home beds of each ownership type; PPHA beds are not included.

[d]Note that the sizable increase in nursing home beds over the previous year resulted from the creation of the HRF category rather than from true growth in the bed stock.

[e]NA = Not Available.

Table D-7
Bed Supply: South Dakota[a]

	1960	1961	1962	1963	1964	1965	1966	1967	1968	1969	1970	1971	1972	1973	1974
Skilled															
Number	—	—	—	—	—	796	1,050	1,978	2,283	2,437	3,087	3,127	3,191	3,656	3,643
% of Total	—	—	—	—	—	23.4	25.0	45.7	42.9	43.9	51.5	49.9	50.1	53.7	53.8
% Increase	—	—	—	—	—	—	31.9	88.4	15.4	6.7	26.7	1.3	2.0	15.5	-0.4
Intermediate	beds in nursing homes and homes for the aged														
Number						2,609	3,151	2,346	3,039	3,117	2,912	3,136	3,176	3,146	3,131
% of Total						76.6	75.0	54.3	57.1	56.1	48.5	50.1	49.9	46.3	46.2
% Increase						—	20.8	-25.5	29.5	2.6	-6.6	7.7	1.3	-0.9	-0.5
Total															
Number	2,511	3,126	3,381	3,506	4,142	3,405	4,201	4,324	5,322	5,554	5,999	6,263	6,367	6,802	6,774
% Increase Beds	—	24.5	8.2	3.7	18.1	—	23.4	2.9	23.1	4.4	8.0	4.4	1.7	6.8	-0.4
Beds per 100 Aged	3.49	4.28	4.57	4.67	5.45	4.42	5.39	5.54	6.74	6.94	7.50	7.64	7.67	8.20	8.06
% Increase Beds/100 Aged	—	22.6	6.8	2.2	16.7	—	21.9	2.8	21.7	3.0	8.1	1.9	0.4	6.9	-1.7
65+ Pop. (in 1,000s)	72	73	74	75	76	77	78	78	79	80	80	82	83	83	84
% Increase 65+ Pop.	—	1.4	1.4	1.4	1.3	1.3	1.3	0	1.3	1.3	0	2.5	1.2	0	1.2
Supervised Personal Care															
Number	—	—	—	—	—	737	636	585	516	648	634	587	590	657	592
% Increase	—	—	—	—	—	—	-13.7	-8.0	-11.8	25.6	-2.2	-7.4	0.5	11.4	9.9
Beds per 100 Aged	—	—	—	—	—	0.96	0.82	0.75	0.65	0.81	0.79	0.72	0.71	0.79	0.70
Proprietary Nursing[b] Home Beds															
Number	NA[c]	NA	NA	NA	NA	NA	NA	1,149	1,715	1,878	2,074	2,108	2,425	2,703	2,723
% of Total	—	—	—	—	—	—	—	26.6	32.2	33.8	34.6	33.7	38.1	39.7	40.2
% Increase	—	—	—	—	—	—	—	—	49.3	9.5	10.4	1.6	15.0	11.5	0.7
Nonprofit Voluntary Nursing[b] Home Beds															
Number	NA	NA	NA	NA	NA	NA	NA	3,135	3,567	3,636	3,885	4,115	3,942	4,099	4,051
% of Total	—	—	—	—	—	—	—	72.5	67.0	65.5	64.8	65.7	61.9	60.3	59.8
% Increase	—	—	—	—	—	—	—	—	13.8	1.9	6.8	5.9	4.2	4.0	-1.2

Public[b] Nursing Home Beds

Number	NA	NA	NA	NA	NA	NA	NA	40	40	40	40	40	0	0
% of Total	—	—	—	—	—	—	—	0.9	0.8	0.7	0.7	0.6	0	0
% Increase	—	—	—	—	—	—	—	—	0	0	0	0	−100.0	0

[a]Figures reflect the number of licensed beds in July of each year with the exception of 1974, for which figures reflect licensed beds as of January.

[b]Figures reflect number of nursing home beds of each ownership type; Supervised Personal Care beds are not included.

[c]NA = Not Available.

Table D-8
Bed Supply: Vermont[b]

	1962	1963	1964	1965	1966	1967	1968	1969	1970	1971	1972	1973	1974
Skilled													
Number	NA[a]	NA	NA	NA	NA	541	514	699	788	1,041	1,046	1,130	843
% of Total	—	—	—	—	—	26.0	25.4	33.0	39.6	47.0	44.3	37.4	27.3
% Increase	—	—	—	—	—	—	-5.0	36.0	12.7	32.1	0.5	8.0	-25.4
Intermediate													
Number	NA	NA	NA	NA	NA	1,538	1,509	1,418	1,201	1,176	1,316	1,888	2,247
% of Total	—	—	—	—	—	74.0	74.6	67.0	60.4	53.0	55.7	62.6	72.7
% Increase	—	—	—	—	—	—	-1.9	-6.0	-15.3	-2.1	11.9	43.5	19.0
Total													
Number	1,747	1,892	NA	NA	2,067	2,079	2,023	2,117	1,989	2,217	2,362	3,018	3,090
% Increase Beds	—	8.3	—	—	—	0.6	-2.7	4.6	-6.0	11.5	6.5	27.8	2.4
Beds per 100 Aged	4.0	4.3	—	—	4.4	4.4	4.2	4.2	4.2	4.6	4.8	6.0	6.1
% Increase Beds/100 Aged	—	7.5	—	—	0	0	-4.6	0	4.2	9.5	4.4	25.0	1.7
65+ Pop. (in 1,000s)	44	44	45	46	47	47	48	50	47	48	49	50	51
% Increase 65+ Pop.	0	0	2.3	2.2	2.1	0	2.1	4.2	-6.0	2.1	2.1	2.0	2.0
Homes for the Aged													
Number	623	670	NA	NA	571	601	589	611	NA	NA	NA	NA	NA
% Increase	—	7.5	—	—	—	5.3	-2.0	3.7	—	—	—	—	—
Beds per 100 Aged	1.4	1.5	—	—	1.2	1.3	1.2	1.2	—	—	—	—	—
Proprietary Nursing Home Beds													
Number	1,591	1,724	NA	NA	1,853	1,854	1,814	1,866	1,663	1,852	2,003	2,614	2,678
% of Total	91.1	91.1	—	—	89.6	89.2	89.7	88.1	83.6	83.5	84.8	86.6	86.7
% Increase	—	8.4	—	—	—	0.1	-2.2	2.9	-10.9	11.4	8.2	30.5	2.4
Nonprofit Nursing Home Beds													
Number	156	168	NA	NA	214	225	209	251	326	365	359	404	412
% of Total	8.9	8.9	—	—	10.4	10.8	10.3	11.9	16.4	16.5	15.2	13.4	13.3
% Increase	—	7.7	—	—	—	5.1	-7.1	20.1	29.9	12.0	-7.8	12.5	2.0

[a]NA = Not Available.
[b]Bed counts reflect censuses as of October in 1962, November in 1963, June in 1966 and 1967, April in 1968, January in 1969 and 1970, November in 1973 and 1974. Census dates for 1964, 1965, 1971, and 1972 could not be ascertained.

Table D-9
Bed Supply: West Virginia

	1960	1961	1962	1963	1964	1965	1966	1967	1968	1969	1970	1971	1972	1973	1974
Nursing Home[a]															
Number of Beds[b]	–	1,355	1,643	1,498	1,532	–	–	–	–	–	1,861	2,151	2,427	2,569	3,170
% Increase[c]	–	–	21.3	–8.8	2.3	3.3	3.3	3.3	3.3	3.3	3.3	15.6	12.8	5.9	23.4
Beds per 100 Aged	–	0.77	0.93	0.84	0.85	–	–	–	–	–	0.96	1.09	1.21	1.27	1.54
% Inc. in Beds per 100 Aged	–	–	20.7	–11.8	1.21	–	–	–	–	–	–	13.5	11.0	4.9	21.2
Personal Care Home[d]															
Number of Beds[b]	–	–	–	–	–	–	–	–	–	–	–	983	975	1,032	998
% Increase[c]	–	–	–	–	–	–	–	–	–	–	–	–	–0.8	5.9	–3.3
Beds per 100 Aged	–	–	–	–	–	–	–	–	–	–	–	0.50	0.49	0.51	0.48

[a]"Nursing Home" is a classification used by the West Virginia State licensing office. This classification today approximates licensed SNF and ICF beds. For earlier years it encompasses homes rendering comparable type care.

[b]Data are on a fiscal-year basis, so that 1961 is actually FY 1962 and 1974 is actually FY 1975.

[c]The percent increase figures for FY 1966 through FY 1971 are average annual rates of growth over that whole period.

[d]There are no figures available for personal care homes for earlier years. There are two ways of estimating how many people were in personal care homes in 1960-1961. Speir (PHS, DHEW, *Characteristics of Nursing Homes and Related Facilities*) indicates that in 1961 there were 392 beds in homes for the aged. The 1960 Census shows 1,976 residents in homes for the aged and dependent not known to have nursing care.

Table D-10
Bed Supply: Wisconsin[a]

	1960	1961	1962	1963	1964	1965
Skilled[b] Care						
Number	NA[e]	NA	NA	NA	19,608	24,096
% of Total	−	−	−	−	91.2	92.0
% Increase	−	−	−	−	−	22.9
Limited Care						
Number	NA	NA	NA	NA	1,901	2,095
% of Total	−	−	−	−	8.8	8.0
% Increase	−	−	−	−	−	10.2
TOTAL						
Number	NA	NA	NA	NA	21,509	26,191
% Increase Beds	−	−	−	−	−	21.8
Beds per 100 Aged	−	−	−	−	5.00	6.00
% Increase Beds/100 Aged	−	−	−	−	−	20.0
65+ Pop. (in 1,000s)	403	413	419	425	432	440
% Increase 65+ Pop.	−	2.5	1.5	1.4	1.7	1.9
Personal Care[c]						
Number	NA	NA	NA	NA	5,815	3,013
% of Total	−	−	−	−	−	−48.2
% Increase	−	−	−	−	1.3	0.7
Proprietary[d] Nursing Home Beds						
Number	7,938	8,790	9,316	10,282	12,064	13,512
% of Total	44	42	42	42	44	46
% Increase	−	10.7	6.0	10.4	17.3	12.0
Nonprofit[d] Vol. Nursing Home Beds						
Number	4,961	6,339	6,494	7,563	8,770	9,104
% of Total	27	30	29	31	32	31
% Increase	−	27.8	2.5	16.5	16.0	3.8
Public[d] Nursing Home Beds						
Number	5,159	5,960	6,375	6,342	6,490	6,588
% of Total	29	28	29	27	24	23
% Increase	−	15.5	7.0	−0.5	2.3	1.5

[a]Bed counts reflect censuses as of July 1 for each year, 1964-1974. Census dates for 1960 through 1963 could not be ascertained.

[b]This category is comprised of beds in nursing homes licensed as "skilled care" facilities and beds in county homes designated as "skilled care" facilities. Some of these are equivalent to SNF level beds, others to ICF level beds.

[c]This category is comprised of beds in nursing homes licensed as "personal care" homes and beds in county homes designated as "personal care" facilities.

[d]Figures include personal care as well as skilled and limited care beds.

[e]NA = Not Available.

1966	1967	1968	1969	1970	1971	1972	1973	1974
27,269	29,979	32,153	34,387	36,261	38,968	40,363	42,289	48,409
93.7	95.4	96.3	96.8	96.4	97.6	97.2	98.1	97.8
13.2	9.9	7.3	7.0	5.5	7.5	3.6	4.8	14.5
1,826	1,443	1,224	1,127	1,369	962	1,168	833	1,097
6.3	4.6	3.7	3.2	3.6	2.4	2.8	1.9	2.2
12.8	−21.0	−15.2	−7.9	21.5	−29.7	21.4	−28.7	31.7
29,095	31,422	33,377	35,514	37,630	39,930	41,531	43,122	49,506
11.1	8.0	6.2	6.4	6.0	6.1	4.0	3.8	14.8
6.52	6.95	7.30	7.67	8.00	8.28	8.51	8.71	9.80
8.3	7.7	4.3	5.5	3.9	3.8	2.4	2.4	12.6
446	452	457	463	471	482	488	495	505
1.4	1.4	1.1	1.3	1.7	2.3	1.2	1.4	2.0
2,372	2,272	2,100	1,567	1,921	2,010	1,704	1,875	1,443
−21.3	−4.2	−7.6	−25.4	22.6	9.4	−15.2	10.0	−23.0
0.5	0.5	0.5	0.3	0.4	0.4	0.3	0.4	0.3
14,719	15,007	16,772	16,604	19,283	21,357	21,876	22,506	24,081
47	44	47	44	48	50	50	50	44
8.9	2.0	11.8	−1.0	16.1	10.8	2.4	2.9	7.0
9,943	10,659	10,902	11,452	11,550	11,826	12,513	13,336	12,593
31	31	30	30	29	28	29	29	23
9.2	7.2	2.3	5.0	0.9	2.4	5.8	6.6	5.6
6,805	8,601	8,378	9,600	9,458	9,497	9,124	9,433	18,089
22	25	23	26	23	22	21	21	33
3.3	26.4	−2.6	14.6	−1.5	0.4	−3.9	3.4	91.8

**Appendix E:
State Sample Selection
Criteria**

Since we desired an understanding of the dynamics and subtleties of nursing home expansion, we sought a sample of states with diverse experience. It was first of all essential to work with a group of states that represented a wide range of rates in nursing home growth. Thus, the primary selection criterion was the rate at which nursing home utilization (number of nursing home residents per 100 elderly population) increased over the study period, 1964-1974. Using this criterion, all fifty states were divided into quintiles. From this it was decided to choose states from the first, third, and fifth quintiles. Other selection criteria were then applied to insure diversity in state characteristics known or hypothesized to influence the level of nursing home growth:

Initial Utilization Level. Given the need or demand for nursing home care in a state, pressures for expansion, it appeared, would be greater the lower the level of use at the outset of the period. We consequently sought to include states which had both high and low rates of nursing home utilization prior to 1964.

Program Expansiveness. Given the level of demand for bed increases, state policies, we reasoned, would probably be most conducive to growth in those states which generally have expansive medical care and social welfare programs. We therefore sought states with a range of levels of expansiveness in their Medicaid programs.

Extensiveness of Elderly Poverty. The level of per capita income and the extent of poverty also have been hypothesized to affect demands for nursing home care. We therefore determined to include a combination of states which had both proportionately large and small poor elderly populations.

Regional Breadth. The most marked regional patterns in nursing home utilization are the low level of utilization in most southeastern states and the very high utilization levels prevalent in the North Central states. We therefore assumed inclusion of southern states in our sample in an effort to isolate factors responsible for this pattern. However, we also sought to include several other regions, especially the north central region, because of its high level of nursing home use.

Rural/Urban. A number of characteristics of rural states may cause their nursing home demands to differ from those of urban states. These include economic, health, and demographic characteristics of their populations. For this reason we wanted to insure the inclusion of both dominantly rural and dominantly urban/industrial states.

State Size. Although state size has not been hypothesized to influence nursing home demands or supply responses, we desired a sample which would account for a significant proportion of total national nursing home use. For this reason we sought a sample which, while including small rural states, would include at least 30 percent of national nursing home population.

Data by States on Variables Used in Selecting a Sample

Variables. Data on the variables discussed below are presented for all states in table E-1. The figure in parentheses indicates the column of table E-1 in which the variable is located.

(1) Annual Rate of Change of Nursing Home Utilization 1960-1973. This is the primary variable used to discriminate among states in selecting a sample below. As indicated, states were first ranked and then divided into quintiles on the basis of the rate at which the nursing home utilization of the elderly rose between 1960 and 1974. Four states were then selected from each of the first, third, and fifth quintiles on the basis of other characteristics discussed above.

Two points concerning this variable merit attention. First, the focus of this study was principally on the increased *rate* at which nursing homes care has come to be used by the elderly. This is somewhat different from the absolute increase in nursing home use which is due in part simply to increases in the over-sixty-five population. Focusing, as does column 1, on increases in the rate of utilization controls for increases attributable only to changes in the size of the over-sixty-five population. Second, these data refer to average annual increases between 1960 and 1973, rather than between 1964 and 1974, which are the years enclosing the study period. Data, however, were not available for 1974, so the closest year for which data are available, 1973, was used as the final year in developing the table entries. Matters are more complicated around the base year for the study. State data on residents are not available for 1964, but are available from the census for 1960 and from the NCHS Master Facility Inventory for 1967.

The data in table E-2 assisted us in selecting 1960 rather than 1967 as the base year for choosing a sample. These figures indicate that if 1967 were used as a base year, the rapid increases between 1963 and 1967 would be neglected. A distorted representation of the 1964-1974 period would then form the basis for state selection. Although 1960 also is not the base year for the study, it appears to be separated from the base year by a period of lesser significance for the nursing home industry. The meager 1.5 percent annual increase in nursing home beds between 1960 and 1963 suggests that the use of 1960 as a base will yield, for most states, a more accurate impression of 1964-1974 changes than if 1967 data were used. This means that, in calculating growth rates, later-year data from NCHS were contrasted with base-year data from the census. A comparison of data from the two sources for a year when both were available suggested,

Table E-1

Arrangement of States by Quintile of Growth in Nursing Home Utilization and by Other Selected Variables, 1960-1973

	Percent Annual Change in NH Residents as Percentage of 65+ Population	Percent Annual Change in Number of NH Residents 1960-1973	NH Residents as Percentage of the 65+ Population 1960	1973	Population 75+ as a Percentage of 65+ Population	Percent Aged with Incomes below 1.25 × Poverty Level 1970	Ratio of Medicaid Users under 65 to Persons under 65 below Poverty Level 1970	State NH Residents as Percent of National Total
	(1)	(2)	(3)	(4)	(5)	(6)	(7)	(8)
1st Quintile								
Arkansas	12.11	13.67	1.52	6.72	38.3	58.1	.078	1.36
Texas	10.60	12.74	1.84	6.82	36.7	44.8	.085	5.68
South Dakota	10.27	10.89	2.53	9.02	41.8	41.9	.143	0.61
New Mexico	10.22	12.70	1.03	3.65	35.7	44.6	.273	0.22
Louisiana	10.21	12.31	1.26	4.46	34.9	53.2	.122	1.20
Georgia	10.15	12.46	1.83	6.43	36.0	50.0	.280	2.12
Alabama	10.01	12.30	1.14	3.94	36.2	55.2	.103	1.16
Wyoming	9.06	9.64	1.92	5.93	39.4	34.8	.178	0.15
California	8.87	10.49	2.56	7.73	38.6	27.8	1.500	11.18
Kentucky	8.54	9.20	1.74	5.05	38.6	49.5	.372	1.38
Mean	10.00	11.64	1.74	5.98	37.6	46.0	.313	2.51
2nd Quintile								
Colorado	8.20	9.38	2.97	8.27	40.7	32.9	.457	1.31
Oklahoma	8.20	9.46	2.92	8.13	39.0	49.8	.400	2.04
Wisconsin	8.15	8.03	3.68	10.20	39.9	33.6	.576	3.51
South Carolina	7.90	10.15	1.40	3.76	34.4	51.3	.128	0.65
Idaho	7.43	8.71	2.23	5.66	40.6	40.8	.270	0.33
North Dakota	7.26	8.21	3.73	9.28	41.0	36.6	.209	0.53
Tennessee	7.08	8.82	1.41	3.43	36.9	51.1	.163	1.13
Montana	6.97	7.27	2.72	6.53	43.5	37.0	.272	0.38
North Carolina	6.90	9.12	2.02	4.81	35.2	47.4	no data	1.70
Maine	6.77	7.30	2.85	6.68	40.1	37.4	.471	0.66
Mean	7.49	8.65	2.59	6.68	39.1	41.8	.327	1.22

3rd Quintile								
Minnesota	6.51	7.31	4.38	9.94	41.2	36.2	.581	3.37
Mississippi	6.39	7.85	1.44	3.22	36.4	63.3	.096	0.64
Michigan	5.97	6.70	2.86	6.08	38.0	32.1	.554	3.68
Illinois	5.91	6.23	3.16	6.67	38.5	31.5	no data	5.87
Nevada	5.86	10.97	1.86	3.90	31.9	31.9	.408	0.11
Vermont	5.74	5.75	3.69	7.62	40.3	35.7	.707	0.29
Nebraska	5.66	6.00	4.15	8.49	42.5	37.5	.313	1.26
New Jersey	5.56	7.05	2.32	4.69	36.9	25.6	.669	2.74
Indiana	5.45	5.65	3.08	6.14	39.5	35.0	.615	2.44
Utah	5.40	7.69	2.66	5.27	37.9	34.9	.447	0.36
Mean	5.84	7.12	2.96	6.20	38.3	36.4	.488	2.08
4th Quintile								
Kansas	5.38	5.85	3.88	7.67	42.0	38.4	.487	1.70
Ohio	5.28	5.67	3.15	6.15	39.4	33.9	.383	5.04
Missouri	5.26	5.73	2.90	5.65	39.9	41.8	.392	2.62
Connecticut	5.17	6.64	3.95	7.61	39.5	23.1	.810	1.92
Maryland	4.68	7.12	2.87	5.20	35.9	28.6	.771	1.38
Alaska	4.65	6.51	4.20	7.58	29.2	32.4	no Medicaid program	0.04
Washington	4.64	5.57	4.99	9.00	40.6	33.8	.888	2.45
Iowa	4.62	4.53	5.01	9.01	42.7	38.3	.379	2.54
Oregon	4.49	6.15	3.93	6.96	40.1	33.4	.403	1.37
Massachusetts	4.48	5.46	4.10	7.25	40.1	27.0	no data	4.07
Mean	4.86	5.92	3.90	7.21	38.9	33.1	.564	2.31
5th Quintile								
Hawaii	4.44	8.31	3.04	5.35	33.2	26.2	.958	0.22
Pennsylvania	4.35	4.99	2.83	4.92	37.9	32.6	1.110	5.23
Arizona	4.33	9.71	1.89	3.28	33.3	32.0	no Medicaid program	0.49
Florida	3.98	8.91	1.77	2.94	34.6	32.5	.221	2.58
Rhode Island	3.75	4.87	3.62	5.84	38.5	32.3	.849	0.52
Virginia	3.60	5.23	2.48	3.93	36.3	38.9	.192	1.21
Delaware	3.23	8.21	2.07	4.71	38.0	31.7	.680	0.18
New York	3.18	3.90	3.03	4.55	36.5	29.3	1.700	7.30
New Hampshire	2.62	3.73	4.86	6.80	39.3	34.4	.422	0.46
West Virginia	1.61	2.17	1.82	2.24	37.4	49.1	.385	0.36
Mean	3.51	6.00	2.74	4.46	36.5	33.9	.652	1.86
United States[a]	5.03	7.13	2.84	5.39	38.0	38.2	.588	100.00

Sources: Column (a) 1960: Residents—U.S. Bureau of the Census, Census of Population: *1960, Final Report, Inmates of Institutions*, PC(2)-8A (1964), Table 37. Elderly—U.S. Bureau of the Census, *Statistical Abstract of the United States: 1964* (1964), p. 23, 1973: National Center for Health Statistics, unpublished data. Column (2) 1960: Census, *Inmates*, Table 37. 1973: NCHS, unpublished data. Column (3) Residents—Census, Inmates, Table 37. Elderly—Census, *Statistical Abstract*, p. 23. Column (4) NCHS, unpublished data. Column (5) U.S. Bureau of the Census, Census of Population: 1970, Vol. 1, *Characteristics of the Population*, Parts 2-52 (1973), Table 48. Column (6) Ibid., Table 58. Column (7) Users—U.S. Department of Health, Education and Welfare, National Center for Social Statistics, *Numbers of Recipients and Amounts of Payments Under Medicaid and Other Medical Programs Financed From Public Assistance Funds, 1970.* Poverty Data—U.S. Bureau of the Census, Census of Population: 1970, *General Social and Economic Characteristics*, Final Report PC(1)-C1 United States Summary (1972), Column (8) NCHS, unpublished data.

[a]With the exception of column 6, national totals are derived from data on the United States as a whole. Because no U.S. data on the percent of the aged with incomes below 125 percent of the poverty level are available from the 1970 Census, the national total for column 6 is the mean of the state percentages and thus weights each state equally, regardless of population.

Table E-2
Rate of Nursing Home Care Use

	1960^a		1963^b		1967^b
Residents of Nursing Homes and Related Facilities	470		491		756
Annual Rate of Increase		1.5		11.4	

[a]Source: U.S. Bureau of the Census, *1960, Final Report, Census of Inmates of Institutions,* Table 7.

[b]Source: U.S. Bureau of the Census, *Statistical Abstract of the United States,* 1972, p. 75.

however, that this would have virtually no distorting effects on the calculated rates of increase.

The 1973 data are based on the NCHS figures for total residents in "nursing care and related homes," a category which includes "nursing care homes," "personal care homes" (with and without nursing), and "domiciliary care homes." The 1960 data are based on the census figures for total residents in "homes for the aged and dependent," a category which includes "homes known to have nursing," and "homes not known to have nursing."

The census definition of "homes for the aged and dependent" is too vague to allow for a detailed comparison of its criteria and those of the NCHS definition of "nursing care and related homes," but both definitions seem to include all facilities providing care below the level of hospitalization but above simple room and board. The similarity of the data collected using the two definitions strongly suggests that they are comparable.

The 1970 Census presents data on conditions found on April 1, 1970. The 1969 and 1971 NCHS Master Facility Censuses present data on conditions found in September, and in October and November of 1969 and 1971, respectively. A comparison by state of the census figures and adjusted NCHS figures (the 1969 figure for each state plus one-quarter of the differences between the 1969 and 1971 figures for that state) produced a correlation coefficient of .99862. The 1970 Census national total of 927,514 residents is 1.5 percent higher than the adjusted NCHS total of 913,857 residents.

Because the definition used in 1970 by the Bureau of the Census and the one used in 1969 and 1971 by the NCHS produced almost identical figures and because the definition used by the Bureau of the Census in 1960 was identical to the one it used in 1970, and the one used by the NCHS in 1973 was the same as the one it used in 1971, the combination of 1960 Census data with 1973 NCHS data seemed justified.

(2) Annual Rate of Change of Nursing Home Populations—1960-1973. These figures indicate the annual rate at which the number of nursing home residents increased over the period 1960 to 1973. These figures are (for all but two states) larger than those of column 1 because they are not deflated by the increasing number of persons over sixty-five. The differences between the column 2 and column 1 figures are greatest in those states where the elderly population has risen rapidly—for example, in Florida and Arizona.

(3)(4) Nursing Home Residents as a Percentage of the Population Aged 65 and Older: 1960 and 1973.

(5) Persons Aged 75 and Older as a Percentage of the Population Aged 65 and Older.

(6) Percentage of Elderly Persons/Households with Incomes Less than 125 Percent of the Poverty Level, 1970.

(7) Ratio of Nonelderly Medicaid Users to the Nonelderly Poverty Population: 1970. As indicated above, we hypothesized that states with generally expansive medical care programs would be more likely to meet the nursing home needs of their populations than would "less generous" states. Nursing home program generosity may be perceived directly in eligibility criteria, reimbursements, and other nursing home policy. However, we lacked data on such program characteristics at the outset of our effort. Furthermore, we sought an expansiveness measure which was not directly dependent on nursing home policy. Consequently, we chose a measure of the general expansiveness of the state Medicaid program. The figures cited here show how effective the state programs were in meeting the medical care needs of their poor and near poor nonelderly populations.

(8) State Nursing Home Population as a Percentage of National Nursing Home Population: 1970.

Identification of Sample States

First Quintile: States with Unusually High Utilization Increase. As a group these states had unusually low utilization levels in 1960 and had relatively extensive populations of elderly poor and relatively restricted Medicaid programs in 1970. The states we initially selected from this quintile are: Alabama, California, South Dakota, and Texas.

When characterized by several of the variables and compared with all states in the first quintile, these four states are distributed in the following patterns.

Table E-3
States with Unusually High Utilization Increases

	Initial Level of Utilization	Extent of Elderly Poverty	Expansiveness of Medicaid Program
High	South Dakota California	Alabama	California
Medium	Texas	Texas South Dakota	
Low	Alabama	California	Texas Alabama South Dakota

Third Quintile: States with Moderate Utilization Increases. As a group these states not only experienced moderate utilization increases but also are close to the mid-point of the ranges of the other variables considered. Nonetheless, within the group of ten states there is considerable diversity along these variables. Much of this, however, results from the inclusion of Mississippi. It is fairly typical of southern states in extent of poverty, restrictiveness of program, and initial (1960) utilization level but differs from the others in having a moderate (6.39), rather than high, annual rate of utilization increase.

The states initially selected from this quintile are: Minnesota, Mississippi, New Jersey, and Vermont.

Included are rural and urban states. When characterized by several of the table E-1 variables and compared with the other third-quintile states, the four sample states are distributed in the following way:

Table E-4
States with Moderate Utilization Increases

	Initial Level of Utilization	Extent of Elderly Poverty	Expansiveness of Medicaid Program
High	Minnesota Vermont	Mississippi	Minnesota Vermont New Jersey
Medium		Minnesota Vermont	
Low	Mississippi New Jersey		

Fifth Quintile: States with Very Low Increases in Utilization. As a group the states with the lowest rates of utilization increase had relatively little poverty and relatively expansive Medicaid programs. The low growth they experienced thus cannot be traced to generally restrictive programs or to high initial utilization rates, since on average their utilization in 1960 was moderate for that period. The combination of moderate initial utilization rates and low rates of increase results in these states having the lowest end-of-period utilization—4.46 percent of their elderly populations. As in the other quintiles, there is considerable diversity by other state characteristics.

The states initially selected from the low-growth quintile are: Arizona, New York, Virginia, and West Virginia. The distribution of selected states when compared with other states in the fifth quintile is shown below.

Table E-5
States with Very Low Increases in Utilization

	Initial Level of Utilization	Extent of Elderly Poverty	Expansiveness of Medicaid Program[a]
High	New York	West Virginia	New York
Medium		Virginia	
Low	West Virginia Arizona Virginia	Arizona New York	Virginia West Virginia

[a]Arizona did not have a Medicaid program in 1970 and thus is excluded from this column.

Final Selection

Table E-6 covers all sample states and shows how, when compared with all fifty states, they are distributed according to the selection variables. The percentage of U.S. nursing home residents who resided in individual states' homes in 1973 are indicated in the first column.

It is evident that the included states provide considerable diversity along the listed variables.

Table E-6
Distribution of Sample States by Selected Variables

	Rate of Utilization Increase		Initial Level of Utilization	Extent of Elderly Poverty	Expansiveness of Medicaid Program
High	Alabama	1.16	Minnesota	Alabama	California
	California	11.18	Vermont	Mississippi	New York
	South Dakota	.61		West Virginia	
	Texas	5.60			
Medium	Minnesota	3.37	California	South Dakota	Vermont
	Mississippi	.64	New York	Texas	Minnesota
	New Jersey	2.74	South Dakota	Virginia	New Jersey
	Vermont	.29	Virginia		
Low	Arizona	.49	Alabama	Arizona	Alabama
	New York	7.30	Arizona	California	Mississippi
	Virginia	1.21	Mississippi	Minnesota	South Dakota
	West Virginia	.36	New Jersey	New Jersey	Texas
			Texas	New York	Virginia
			West Virginia	Vermont	West Virginia

Index

Index

About the Author

Burton David Dunlop is Senior Research Associate at the Urban Institute, Washington, D.C., where he is engaged in gerontological research with a focus on long-term care. Dr. Dunlop received the Ph.D. as a Ford Foundation Fellow at the University of Illinois. He has published in the *Journal of Chronic Diseases* and has written papers for or participated in a number of task forces, legislative hearings, continuing education programs, symposia, and panels concerned with long-term care.